Praise for *Screen-Smart Parenting*

"As a parent who lives much of my life online and is at the same time concerned about my children's media use, this is the book I've been waiting for. Here is a nonjudgmental, well-informed voice ringing out from the cacophony of anti-screen hysteria. Dr. Gold spells out in crystal-clear terms how we can help kids build the tech savvy they need to become good digital citizens. Most of all, she has helped me understand that in order to address the concerns many of us share about children's technology use, parents need to develop healthy digital lives ourselves."
—*Amy Shearn, parent and novelist*

"An essential read for any parent or caretaker concerned about the effects of our children being constantly plugged in. Dr. Gold provides invaluable information and guidance, and helps us feel calmer and more comfortable in these heretofore uncharted waters."
—*Debra Messing, actress and mother*

"Just as our mothers and fathers worried about too much TV, today's parents worry about their children getting lost in cyberspace. . . . With *Screen-Smart Parenting*, Dr. Jodi Gold has provided the milestone book that will give important insights to every parent."
—*From the Foreword by Tory Burch, CEO, designer, and mother of three*

"No one understands the digital landscape and its complex presence in our children's lives better than Jodi Gold. This book is a 'must read' for all parents who want to protect their children while still giving them access to all of the benefits technology has to offer. Dr. Gold's realistic approach to navigating the cyberculture is invaluable—she gives easy-to-follow and commonsensical advice. As parents, many of us are new to the digital world, while our children are naturals. This guide gives spot-on strategies for closing that gap and making the whole family's approach to technology effortless."
—*Holly Phillips, MD, general internist and CBS News Medical Contributor*

"This book is so great! As parents of a second and a fifth grader, it is challenging and, honestly, scary to always be on top of what content they are accessing, whom they are communicating with, and for how long. Dr. Gold provides practical tools to help us establish digital rules and enforce them consistently. Her writing style is easy to read and digest—it is extremely personable and never judgmental . . . We will definitely refer back to *Screen-Smart Parenting* often as our daughters grow."
—*Lisa and Steve Freedman, parents*

"Dr. Gold teaches you everything you need to know about what your kids are doing online, how it may affect their development, and what you can do about it. She reviews just about every form of digital media your kids may experience and brings you up to date so you can speak their language. Great tips are provided on managing screen time at all ages."
—*Mitch Prinstein, PhD, Distinguished Professor and Director of Clinical Psychology, University of North Carolina at Chapel Hill*

"Dr. Gold gives advice that's clear, practical, and trustworthy. Every parent should have this book to guide them in making decisions so that their children—from newborns to teens—can reap the benefits of technology while avoiding the pitfalls. I am buying extra copies of this book for my sons, who are both raising young kids."
—*Peg Dawson, EdD, coauthor of* Smart but Scattered

"Dr. Jodi Gold has written the definitive guide to one of the most challenging issues facing parents today: raising kids in a digital age. Drawing on her wealth of experience as a mother and psychiatrist, Dr. Gold provides parents with a blueprint on how to cultivate wise media use at every stage of a child's development. Thoughtful, well researched, and fun to read, this is a book that all parents should have at the top of their reading list. Urgently needed and extremely practical, it is a godsend."
—*Ellen Braaten, PhD, author of* Bright Kids Who Can't Keep Up

"Dr. Gold provides a comprehensive framework that parents can rely on as they face this new, dynamic, and critical parenting challenge of our time."
—*Karen L. Bierman, PhD, Child Study Center and Department of Psychology, The Pennsylvania State University*

SCREEN-SMART PARENTING

screen-smart parenting

How to Find Balance and Benefit in Your Child's Use of Social Media, Apps, and Digital Devices

Jodi Gold, MD

Foreword by Tory Burch

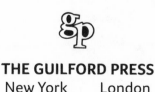

THE GUILFORD PRESS
New York   London

© 2015 The Guilford Press
A Division of Guilford Publications, Inc.
72 Spring Street, New York, NY 10012
www.guilford.com

Printed in the United States of America

This book is printed on acid-free paper.

Last digit is print number: 9   8   7   6   5   4   3   2   1

Library of Congress Cataloging-in-Publication Data

Gold, Jodi.
    Screen-smart parenting : how to find balance and benefit in your child's use
of social media, apps, and digital devices / by Jodi Gold.
        pages cm
    Includes bibliographical references and index.
    ISBN 978-1-4625-1553-0 (paperback)   ISBN 978-1-4625-1794-7 (hardcover)
    1. Internet and children.   2. Parenting.   3. Social media.   I. Title.
HQ784.I58G65 2015
649′.1—dc23

                                                                2014022753

The names, characteristics, and details of individuals described and quoted
in this book have been changed to protect their privacy.

To Mitch, Jackson, Carter, and Samantha—
thank you for your love and support

Foreword

Like most people, I read a lot of parenting books after I had my three boys. These books help parents understand and recognize the different milestones that mark their children's growth. None of the child development books I read covered digital technology, a pervasive influence in the world today.

Just as our mothers and fathers worried about too much TV, today's parents worry about their children getting lost in cyberspace. We all wonder if technology will diminish their intellectual curiosity and if interest in digital games will supersede interest in real-life interaction. Safety and privacy are also an enormous concern. I always went back and forth about the age at which I would allow my children to engage with digital devices and social media.

With *Screen-Smart Parenting*, Dr. Jodi Gold has provided the milestone book that will give important insights to every parent. Dr. Gold understands what it means to raise children in a world that is so different from the one in which she grew up, but as a physician and psychiatrist specializing in children and adolescents, she has an advantage over most parents. Her advice is to focus on what's developmentally appropriate, and to pay attention to the way our children interact with social and digital media. It's important not to completely deny access, but there should be balance and moderation. Our children need to know how to navigate this new world—and, as parents, we need to know how to guide them and make the Internet a source of positive experiences.

Screen-Smart Parenting provides a blueprint for parents today. Dr. Gold has mapped out the digital milestones and given families the tools they need to help them help their children stay on the track. In a time when there is always a new device or platform just around the corner, Dr. Gold's book is a relevant and timely addition to any parent's library.

TORY BURCH
CEO and designer
Mother of three

Acknowledgments

Screen-Smart Parenting has been like a fourth child to me. It has been a labor of love, sweat, and tears. I never would have had the strength and courage to write this book without the support of my parents, Rochelle and Bob, who instilled in me a genuine respect and awe for technology and innovation and taught me the grit and perseverance needed to complete a book.

My family has been endlessly patient as I headed off to Le Pain Quotidien to write yet another chapter. Thank you to Mitch Jacaruso, who has never faltered in his belief in me and picked up the pieces of our lives as this project unfolded. Jackson, Carter, and Samantha have been and always will be my inspiration. They helped me realize the critical need to chart a purposeful course through the digital world. I also thank Tom and Stephanie Card, who are my artistic and creative inspirations.

I never planned or intended to write this book. John Walkup jump-started the process and put the project into motion. Kitty Moore and Chris Benton of The Guilford Press are the best editors and mentors I could have asked for. Chris and Kitty made the process reasonable, fun, and efficient. I never would have started or finished this project without them. I miss their endless e-mails and calls. Thank you.

Tory Burch took time out of her busy life to lend support to this project. She is a role model to us all. Samantha Boardman has been encouraging and helpful throughout this entire journey. Liz Keough has been a true friend, sounding board, and editor.

Sharlene Leong, Lola Seaton, Sarah Safaie, Carrie Parker, Carmen Rodriguez, and Megan Buckley have provided invaluable assistance. Anne Mansfield told me to "lean in" and made me feel not so crazy about embarking on this project. Marie Will helped me to get back on track early in the process. Odette Muskin taught me how to bring technology into nursery school. Thank you to Susan Villari, my coeditor on my first book, *Just Sex: Students Rewrite the Rules on Sex, Violence, Activism, and Equality.* Producing that book was a long and arduous process, but it gave me the skills and confidence to even consider this project.

Thanks to Paula Berry at Common Sense Media, who truly believed in and fought for me; Lucy Baker and the whole team at The Guilford Press; Suzanne Williams and Laura Rossi, an amazing publicity team; and Chelsea Rogers and Jayson Jacobs, for sticking with me as I tried to carve out my own digital footprint.

Thank you to my teachers and mentors—Dr. Ted Shapiro, Dr. Margaret Hertzig, and Dr. Betsy Auchincloss—for bringing me to Cornell and teaching me what it means to be a good physician and psychiatrist; Dr. Catherine Birndorf, whose mentorship has been invaluable in this process; Ed and Robin Berman, for their honest advice; and Holly Phillips and Debra Messing, who took the time to read and critique the manuscript.

I am indebted to the collective wisdom of my friends and colleagues who contributed vignettes, thoughts, and opinions: Heba Abedin, Julie Ader, Bonne Altman, Cindy Dobbs, Kiara Ellozy, Pete and Jen Evans, Jennifer Feldman, Lisa and Steve Freedman, Julie Friedland, Liz Gateley, Estelle Gehrig, Lori Gleeman, Risa Gold, Jen Hoine, Lara Oboler and Lou Jaffe, Sarah Klagsbrun, Stacy Kuhn, Jessica Lawrence, Adrienne Lederer, Shari Minsky, Lesley Perlman, Mark Rabiner and Avi Pemper, Michelle Rubel, Carly Snyder, Amy Silverman, Regan Stanger, Renee Sullivan, Wendy Turchin, Lisa Van Houten, Janie Vance, Robin Wallace, Kara Wyatt, Christy Yarbro, Felice Yestion, and Soo Mi Young.

Contents

III. ONE SIZE DOES NOT FIT ALL

Purchasers can download and print select practical tools
from this book at *www.guilford.com/gold-forms*.

Introduction

Throw Away the Rule Book

For thousands of years, we have relied on our parents, grandparents, aunts, and uncles for parenting advice. While we often get advice that we don't want and didn't ask for, we instinctively turn to what our parents might have done. Recently, I have found myself asking the following questions:

"When did my parents reward my good behavior with apps?"

"How did I finish my homework while texting, chatting, tweeting, and posting?"

"How old was I when my parents gave me my first smartphone?"

"How did my parents choose which Disney series to download, and which role-playing video game (RPG) was acceptable to play?"

"How did my parents keep my sister and me safe and protected from cyberbullying and sexting?"

"How did my parents help us manage our digital footprint and instill in us the tenets of good digital citizenship?"

"How did my parents help me balance the need to be digitally connected with the need for real play and real human interaction?"

Wait! I grew up in the 1970s and '80s, and my parents were awesome, but they didn't face any of these dilemmas. I was born before the digital revolution. I am what is now called a "digital immigrant." Technology is not my first language. I have learned it and embraced it, and it now runs much of my life, but I'm not completely fluent. I speak "technology" or "Digitalese" with an accent. If I am keeping track properly, my 9-year-old and 7-year-old sons are the youngest members of the iGeneration, the millennials, or the "app generation"—born since the inception of the Internet. My 5-year-old daughter, born in 2008, is a "Digitod." The Internet is ancient history for her generation. She was born after the iPhone and following the touch-screen revolution.

Technology has changed since you were a kid. In fairness, technology is always changing, and every generation of mothers and fathers faces a different landscape from their parents. My father never tired of telling me that his family was one of the first in Winnipeg to own a television. He and his brother sat for hours watching the "Indian-head" test pattern before there was any real programming. From the 1950s to the '80s technology advanced at the speed of sound, but today we are experiencing progress at the speed of light.

There is an ongoing intellectual debate about whether we drive technology (instrumentalism) or whether it drives us (determinism). Sigmund Freud promoted the concept that our early childhood experiences shape who we are as adults. That is not to say that we can't reshape who we are, but there is no escaping your childhood completely. This is also true when you are parenting. The problem here is that no one has any direct experience with growing up with interactive digital technology. I suspect that our kids will have it a bit easier when they grow up. They will, at least, have experienced childhood in the digital era, from which they can draw parenting tools. Today, no one has any real personal experience helping parents figure out whether toddlers should use the "iPotty" or learn to read on a tablet. No one can say definitively when children should get their first smartphone or sign up for Instagram. How do you help your preteen daughter balance her changing body with the pressures of managing her online identity? How do you help your teenage son manage the demands of high school with the constant intrusions of games, messages, and Instagram?

You and your usual sources are equally lacking in experience on how to parent with digital technology. Unfortunately, the "experts" don't offer much help here either. There is burgeoning research in this area, but limited longitudinal studies. Even studies that have followed kids since the '90s are somewhat outdated at this point. A lot of the early research was fearful and pessimistic. It mostly focused on passive television watching, and there hasn't been much time to focus on interactive digital technology.

My friends and my family repeatedly asked me why I embarked on this project when I have a full-time job and three kids. I decided to embark on this project because as a parent and as a child and adolescent psychiatrist, I wanted to develop a more thoughtful approach to parenting with digital technology. There is so much fear about the digital age. When I tell friends and colleagues about the book, the first response is usually a fearful one: "Are you going to tell parents how to keep their kids safe?" or "Is there any chance that our kids will grow up to have meaningful relationships?" You can run, but you can't hide from the digital age. It is here to stay, so I wanted to develop a more fearless approach where we embrace it and control it so we are not controlled by it.

I've seen mind-boggling benefits accrue to kids who are digital natives, as well as disadvantages, both in my office and at home—some of them completely unexpected. I wanted to combine the collected knowledge of pediatrics, psychiatry, and parenting to answer the questions we digital immigrants ask and to start a constructive dialogue about how we can get the full benefit of this "new" technology for our kids while minimizing any downsides.

I routinely get calls from parents asking if their child is ready for an iPhone and whether it is safe for the child to join Instagram and play Call of Duty. As I sit at Le Pain Quotidien (a New York Belgian-bakery franchise) finishing up the book, all I have to do is listen to people at the neighboring tables to hear the questions. On my right, a young couple Googles "recommended screen times" for toddlers, while their 18-month-old baby sits in the high chair pinching and swiping his parents' other iPhone. On my left, two teenage girls sit facing each other, feverishly texting and laughing while looking at their phones. They are interacting with each other in a way that even the *Jetsons* and the sci-fi movies couldn't have dreamed up when I was growing up in the 1980s. Unfortunately, there is no parenting playbook for each new update and innovation. We are suspicious of SnapChat and fearful of the epidemic of sexting and unprepared for what comes next. Parents, educators, and physicians are in a constant state of "catch-up." We want rules but there are no rules. The goal of this book is to help you develop a thoughtful, systematic approach to digital technology with rules, guidelines, and open communication in place as early as possible.

As with any other parenting issue, our approach needs to be developmentally appropriate. What is appropriate for a 12-year-old may not be for a 9-year-old. When is it OK for your son to start playing World of Warcraft? At what age can your daughter be trusted with the responsibility and privilege of her own smartphone? Throughout this book, I encourage you to rely on your own instincts and your intimate knowledge of your children. You know your family best, and you know the values and customs underlying your family's culture. Trust them to guide you.

Of course you'll also want to know what the research has to say. I offer the scientific evidence that we do have, and when there isn't research, I try to make recommendations based on my teaching and clinical experience. The hope is that your children will develop online resilience and a healthy evolving digital footprint that promotes self-expression, not self-destruction.

A lot of earlier research warned of an anticipated digital divide between rich and poor—the idea that poor kids have less access to digital technology and this will hold them back and keep them in poverty. The "digital divide" research has already changed in the last 5 years, with more computers in classrooms and the smartphone revolution. A recent Northwestern University study found that lower-income families had more devices than families with incomes over $100,000 per year. The current concern is not about access but about usage. If lower-income kids are accessing the Internet with smartphones and not computers, will they be able to create online or only consume? In the early 2000s, researchers were concerned that social networking would replace "real" friendships with online strangers. With the pervasiveness of social media and the Internet, the issue now is how you can best connect with your "real-life" friends in a virtual world.

Our parents can't help us here, and the research keeps on changing. So what do we do now?

Since your parents and the researchers are of little help, we need to go back to the drawing board and develop an upgraded parenting model. We break down this journey into three steps:

1. Figure out your parenting style and family culture. The "rules" by which you parent and the customs followed in your household form the foundation for your children's use of digital technology. You must integrate digital technology into your children's life in a relatively seamless way that is consistent with your family culture, values, and rules. For example, you are doomed to failure if you decide that your 10-year-old son should be limited to 1 hour of gaming per day when your spouse plays Angry Birds for hours and hours. Restricting your 15-year-old daughter's TV time to 2 hours when the TV has been on in the background of your home since her birth could be setting yourself up for conflict. In Chapter 1, I take you through the process of discovering the roots of your parenting, defining your own parenting style, and then candidly assessing your family's technology diet. The ultimate goal is to consider what kind of relationship you have with technology and what kind of relationship you wish to model for your family in the future.

2. Understand the digital landscape. It's important to understand the developmental evolution of the use of digital technology: what happens at what age. It's also essential to get a feel for how digital technology is actually used today by children and adolescents. The entire basis of this book is developmental. That is, all of my analyses and recommendations are founded in an understanding of the developmental goals and milestones of different ages. This developmental model of digital parenting will examine how technology supports growth and what specific issues you need to address at each stage of your child's life. We examine the research on how technology affects your child's development in Chapter 2 and take a tour of the broader digital landscape in Chapter 3. In Chapter 4, I introduce the hot topics that monopolize conversations among parents—everything from the iBlankie to the proverbial 5 minutes of Facebook fame. Then in Part II of this book you'll find chapters about different age groups, each of which explains how digital technology intersects with what your child needs to achieve during those years and how you can promote technology as a tool to support, not hinder, healthy development. In Chapter 11, we take a more sophisticated look at children who need more attention and parental involvement and may exhibit red flags for attention-deficit/hyperactivity disorder (ADHD), anxiety, and depression. These "orchid" children may need extra care and modified digital parameters.

3. Create a family technology plan and family media rules to ensure that technology has a positive impact on your child's development. The subject of rules will come up over and over in this book, with specifics pertaining to different developmental ages in the chapters in Part II. While I'll advocate a few hard-and-fast dos and don'ts, for the most part it's your family and your rules. I will encourage you to be honest with yourself and the reality of your own tech use—which of course you model for your children every day. I will help you think through your own values, beliefs, and customs so you can apply them to your family technology plan. The concluding chapter provides guidelines for putting everything you've read in the book into your personalized family technology plan. I strongly suggest you take the time to formulate a plan for your family. It's the only way to chart an intentional course through this wide-open frontier. With a family technology plan and an understanding of the shifting digital landscape, your family can make the best possible use of digital technology and remain adept, smart, safe users of the most exciting tools the world has ever known.

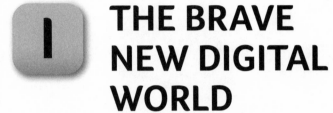

THE BRAVE NEW DIGITAL WORLD

1 Understanding Your Family's Digital Habitat

Cultivating Online Resilience and Digital Citizenship

Lori was the first of my "mom friends" to respond to my request for help. I had e-mailed several moms whom I respect to get their thoughts, worries, and ideas about raising kids in the digital era. Lori is an Ivy League–educated woman who had left her high-powered law firm to be a full-time stay-at-home mother after the birth of her second child, Madeline. She takes her job thoughtfully and seriously.

Lori sent me a three-page (no joke) e-mail on the evils of technology. She explained that her children preferred beautifully illustrated hardcover storybooks and played old-fashioned board games. Madeline is 5, and Jake is 7. She tries to limit their technology as much as possible. While writing this long e-mail, she received a delivery for her 2013 Christmas cards. She opened the box and, much to her dismay, realized that her daughter was holding an iPad in their perfectly posed family portrait.

She was completely aghast. She had defined her family culture by its lack of devices and technology, yet the iPad was front and center and in front of the Christmas tree. Lori is a very funny and self-aware mother, and the irony was not lost on her. She told me to dismiss the three-page e-mail on the evils of technology. It was time, she said, to face the reality that digital technology was fully integrated into her family's life.

She sent back the cards to the company and had the iPad "Photoshopped" out of the picture, but she also began to reassess her dogmatic approach to digital technology. Lori lamented to me that her strict rules had blinded her to the fact that her husband and children were fascinated and intrigued by the innovations of digital technology. Lori took her blinders off and realized that it wasn't only her children who were preoccupied with technology. The evening after the Christmas card fiasco, she was looking for her husband to discuss the new holiday cards. She opened the bathroom door to find her husband, a powerful Wall Street investment banker, curled up in a corner, engrossed in the über-popular game Clash of Clans. She asked him what he was doing, and he explained that he was hiding from the kids (and her) so they wouldn't see him playing the game. Both Lori and I agreed that you can run, but you can't hide, from technology.

Lori, like most parents, is seeking to strike a balance between the "human" and the "virtual." In the 21st century, understanding your family's digital habitat is a critical component to successful parenting.

We all want our children to be happy, successful, and safe. How do we reach this goal? We cannot shield our children from risk (either offline or online) or naively believe that education and knowledge acquisition are the one sure path. It's not rules and restrictions that lead to success and happiness. Adversity is inevitable, and children need to be able to manage it. The cornerstones of adult happiness and success are, it seems, childhood resilience and character. Upon these cornerstones, good citizenship is built, digital and otherwise. **As a psychiatrist, researcher, and mother, I believe that resilience is integral to developing character and citizenship and finding success and happiness both online and offline.**

In his 2009 article "The Science of Success," David Dobbs described what he called dandelion and orchid children. Dandelion children are healthy, or "normal," children with "resilient" genes. They will thrive anywhere, whether it is the metaphorical sidewalk crack or the well-tended garden. In contrast, orchid children will wilt if ignored or maltreated but bloom spectacularly with greenhouse care.[1]

I agree that "resilient genes" play a role in children's ability to manage adversity, but both research and human experience have found that parenting and love can change the course laid out by your genes. **Our**

first digital parenting goal, therefore, is to cultivate online resilience and digital citizenship.

Resilient children turn negative emotions and experiences into positive ones. They successfully navigate adverse situations online not by avoiding them but by being exposed to risk. Overly restrictive parents are less likely to allow for the online mistakes and missteps that are critical to the development of resilience. Online resilience is the foundation for your children's ongoing relationship with technology in every arena, from how to properly use various media platforms to adhering to the tenets of digital citizenship. Children with high levels of self-esteem and confidence are more likely to develop online resilience, while children with more psychological challenges will have more difficulty.[2] (Chapter 11 offers some help to parents whose children have challenges pertinent to digital technology use.)

When I was trying to outline the components of online resilience, I came across Paul Tough's *How Children Succeed*. He eschews the idea that intelligence and high SAT scores lead to success in life. He argues that the qualities that matter most have more to do with character: skills like perseverance, curiosity, conscientiousness, optimism, and self-control.[3] Economists call these "noncognitive skills"; psychologists call it "character," and I will refer to these traits in relation to the digital world as online resilience and digital citizenship. I believe that since your kids will spend more time in the digital world than eating, sleeping, hanging out, or going to school, they need more than real-life resilience. They need online resilience to care for themselves and digital citizenship to care for the world around them.

> You can run, but you can't hide, from digital technology.

Digital citizenship is the most important cyber term that you need to know. Digital citizenship reflects the norms and ethics of responsible and appropriate technology use. For me the term reflects qualities such as kindness, responsibility, conscientiousness, self-control, mindfulness, and altruism. I imagine schoolchildren reciting a pledge like the following after the Pledge of Allegiance:

> Our children need online resilience to take care of themselves and digital citizenship to take care of the world around them.

THE PLEDGE OF THE DIGITAL CITIZEN

I pledge my commitment to upholding the values of digital citizenship. I pledge to take care of my self, others, and my community. I pledge to be mindful and thoughtful of what I say and post online. I pledge to use technology as a tool to improve both myself and my community. I pledge to use the power of the Internet and social media to spread kindness and philanthropy around the world. I pledge to uphold the digital golden rule to "do unto others as I would want them to do unto me."

Digital citizenship has become a tool that schools use to prepare kids for the world of technology. In the United States, there is a national mandate to provide "advanced telecommunication services and information services" to public schools. Digital citizenship is loosely part of the Common Core curriculum. There is no required lesson plan. However, if a school or school district applies for additional funding for technology (called an E-rate grant), it must show proof that it is teaching digital citizenship in its classrooms.[4]

Digital citizenship seems like an obvious positive. There shouldn't be too much to debate. Yet there is a whole literacy genre that includes op-eds, blogs, and books such as *Distracted* and *The Dumbest Generation* that fear technology will usher in a dark age for thought, creativity, and relationships. Many of the most popular movies (e.g., *The Matrix*, *The Terminator*) foretell a dystopian doomsday of brain-dead people controlled by computers. Are we headed into a Brave New World where *1984* comes true in 2015? Obviously I can't answer that question, but the increasing power of technology companies needs to be monitored. So what can we do about it?

We can raise kids who understand digital citizenship . . .

- *We can raise children who can ethically manage Facebook or YouTube or whatever comes next.*
- *We can raise children who are responsible and savvy users.*
- *We can raise politicians who understand the need for separation of powers and separation of technology and state.*

Some examples of how you can promote online resilience and digital citizenship can be found in the box on page 13.

Examples of Ways to Promote Online Resilience

- Talk to your kids about both "good" and "bad" TV.
- Help them to distinguish fantasy from reality on TV, Internet, and social media.
- Challenge the stereotypes they see online and on TV.
- Talking to them about the violence—asking them how the characters might feel.
- Teach them to be critical of advertising images and messages.
- Help them become critical consumers.
- Help them to assess the credibility and authenticity of websites.
- Following them on social media sites.
- Comment in person (not online) about poor choices they or others have made on social media.
- Turn small mistakes online into teachable moments, not punishments.
- Encourage them to apologize for or correct online mistakes.
- Keep open communication, so your kids can talk to you about online mistakes and concerns.

The journey starts at home. It starts with understanding your family culture and your family's digital habitat.

> You want your children to be prepared to head into cyberspace without a babysitter.

BOXERS OR BRIEFS?: DEFINING YOUR FAMILY CULTURE

To create a parenting blueprint that cultivates online resilience and digital citizenship, we must start with an examination of your family culture. Family culture is important because it will drive your family's decisions about technology. It will help you understand and explain your approach to yourselves and to your children. Your family culture consists of who you are as a family inside and outside your broader community. Your ethnicity, religion, education, political views, and values shape your family culture. Each family is different and can't be easily categorized as conservative, liberal, religious, or secular. It is the funny, subtle things that help to define your culture. For instance, what do you call your grandmother? Grandma, Grams, Mamey, Nana, Nonni, Ona, Bubbie, Mum, Mema? Here are some broader questions to get you thinking about your particular family culture.

- How do you celebrate?
- What are your family traditions?
- How do you relax?
- How does your ethnicity and family background affect your family life?
- How does your religion affect your family life?
- How is your family the same as or different from your childhood family?
- What are your goals and priorities for your children?

Your family culture will determine the values that you apply to digital technology. Some families are primed to embrace technology and use it as a tool. Some will be more fearful and distrustful and will treat it as the "enemy." Others will have mixed attitudes. Lori distrusted technology and tried to restrict it, but her husband and children coveted and embraced it. Your family culture should not be driven by technology, but should integrate it in a way that is fun, healthy, and enriching.

In this chapter we explore three elements of family culture that are critical to understanding your family's digital habitat and composing your family technology plan:

- You and your partner's relationship with technology
- Your parenting identity and style
- Your family media consumption category

> Digital technology should be integrated into your family culture in a fun, healthy, and enriching way.

Your Relationship with Technology

Your relationship with technology is a critical part of your family culture. So where do you fit on the technology spectrum? Are you a tech-savvy grown-up? Are you the first to get the upgrade? Do you spend hours figuring out your new gadget, or would you prefer that someone else do it for you? There are no right and wrong answers, but you do need to understand your relationship with technology before you can guide your children. The baby boomers and Generation Xers have been labeled digital immigrants. Cyberspace and digital technology are a second language. Children and young adults born since the technology revolution are called digital natives. They speak digital without an accent. Here are some family culture questions for digital immigrant parents to better understand your relationship with technology.

- What was your first memory of video games? E-mail? Social media?
- Do you embrace or avoid the newest gadget?
- How many TVs do you have in your home?
- Would you consider yourself a heavy, moderate, or light user?
- Do you read the *New York Times* or play Bejeweled when bored?
- On a "date" with your spouse, do you go to the movies or the gym?
- Do you take your phone to the bathroom?
- Do you prefer reading on an e-reader or paper?
- Are you afraid of or excited about your children's digital journey?
- Do you use the Internet regularly or occasionally?
- Are you on Facebook?
- Did you meet your spouse online? Did you ever date online?
- Do you prefer to text or talk?
- Does your job require you to be constantly plugged in?
- Would you consider yourself a healthy digital role model for your children?

Depending on your family culture, you may choose to write, e-mail, text, or keep in your head a list of qualities that define your family. Your list will help you determine whether you embrace, avoid, restrict, or permit.

Coming Clean: Who Are You as a Parent?

Once you have described your family, it is time to reflect on who you are as a parent. When we think about our identity as "Mom" or "Dad," we often describe ourselves in reference to our own parents. Your own memories, regrets, and experiences as children heavily shape who you would like to be as a parent. It doesn't mean that you will turn into your mother or father, but you can't escape them. Whether you realized it or not, the birth of your first child likely triggered your own childhood memories. For the first time in years, you might have found yourself asking how your mother would have handled a situation. Perhaps you didn't give your parents enough credit for their efforts. On the other hand, you may choose to do things quite differently than your parents. For example, you may be strict and limit technology because you perceive that your parents were not "strict enough." For better or worse, your childhood memories and relationship with your parents will heavily determine your parenting identity and choices.

Here is a list of questions to help fine-tune your parental identity:

1. What were your parents' biggest strengths and weaknesses?
2. What influenced your parents' ability to parent? (e.g., divorce, illness, mental health, substance abuse)
3. How did your parents treat your siblings differently?
4. Did your parents have lots of rules and expectations?
5. How did your parents punish you when you did something wrong?
6. Do you have role models for parenting other than your own parents?
7. How would you like to parent similarly and differently than your parents?

These questions are designed to help you formulate a picture of who you are as a parent and where it came from. Questions 1–3 should help you understand your own parents from your current adult vantage point. When trying to decide how to handle digital technology or any other major ingredient in your child's life, it's helpful to know where you might struggle. Those parents who face the most parenting challenges often had an ambivalent or disappointing relationship with their own parents. If this is true for you, then it is important to understand where and how you feel that your parents failed you. You can use their failures to your advantage as you parent your own children in the real and virtual world.

Questions 4 and 5 should paint a picture of your parents' parenting style. If your parents encouraged independence while setting clear expectations, you may feel comfortable giving your children developmentally appropriate freedom to explore and embrace technology. If your parents were critical and demanding, then you may find yourself being generally fearful and restrictive in your parenting. With each real and digital milestone that your child achieves, you may "remember" different things about your childhood and your parents. You may remember your own fear about leaving for summer camp or your own humiliation about disappointing your parents in some way. You should take stock of these memories and moments. If you recall humiliations or disappointments from your own childhood, pay attention. It is these memories and unresolved experiences that may hamper or impact your present-day parental decisions. If you feel like you have mishandled decisions as a parent, think back to your childhood and your own parents for an answer or solution. Be conscious of your sticky memories as a child so you can be mindful in supporting and guiding your own children in a different direction.

The last two questions allow you the opportunity to think forward about how you will use your childhood experiences to positively shape your parenting style. We may not have control over our own childhood experiences, but we can use them to make better parenting decisions for ourselves and our families.

Curfews or Candy?: Defining Your Parenting Style

There is emerging research showing that parenting styles affect your children's media use and their online resilience. Generally, researchers divide parenting styles into four categories: authoritarian, authoritative, permissive, and uninvolved or laissez-faire. More recently, researchers have applied these four categories to digital technology and refer to them as Internet parenting styles. Your general parenting style will undoubtedly be reflected in how you approach and manage technology. Parental warmth and parental control are the two components that mediate digital parenting styles.

Parental warmth or **responsiveness** refers to intentionally fostering individuality and self-regulation. It describes the level to which a parent accommodates and cultivates a child's individual needs.

- A parent with high parental warmth would be more likely to engage children in developing technology rules.
- Parents and children would be more likely to share technology experiences.
- Children would be more likely to share upsetting or shocking online experiences with their parents.

Parental control is linked to restrictions about technology use and clear guidelines about acceptable content.

- Parents with high parental control are more likely to personally supervise or use parental controls and filters to monitor Internet use.
- A parent with high parental control might set non-negotiable technology restrictions.
- Parents with high parental control would focus less on individual needs and more on consistent rules with reliable consequences.

Take this little quiz to find out more about your digital parenting style:

1. My approach to family rules for technology is:
   a. I wouldn't bother.
   b. I would try my best to enforce rules but might have difficulty with follow-through.
   c. I would include my children in the process of developing a family technology plan.
   d. My husband and I will type up clear, consistent rules about when and how technology can be used.

2. Ideally, how would you monitor your child's Internet use?

  a. Wouldn't bother.

  b. Would occasionally look at my child's phone or search history.

  c. Would consistently check my child's texts and quietly follow her on social media sites.

  d. Would install parental controls and filters. I would block inappropriate websites and monitor all activity.

3. Would you allow your son to play online games on school nights?

  a. Of course. What else would he be doing?

  b. Yes. He needs the break, and hopefully he will get his homework done afterwards.

  c. Yes. But he needs to complete his homework and show it to me, and then I am happy to let him play or to play a game with him.

  d. No. Video games are addictive and distracting. He needs to focus on his homework, and he can play games on the weekend.

4. What would you do if you found your daughter sending an inappropriate photo to her boyfriend?

  a. Nothing. It is her private business.

  b. Express concern and discuss what is going on in the relationship.

  c. Express concern about my daughter's self-esteem while contacting the boy's parents to make sure the picture is not forwarded. Then take away her phone for the next few days.

  d. Forbid my daughter from ever seeing the boy again and then take away her phone for the next month.

*If you circled **a** for many questions,* then you may fit into the laissez-faire or uninvolved parenting style. This style is self-explanatory, and it is unlikely that laissez-faire parents are reading this book. *Laissez-faire parenting is linked to poor self-esteem and less resilience in children. It is also the least common style of parenting.*

*If you answered **b** to two or more of these questions,* then you likely fall into the permissive parenting category. Permissive parents often have a high level of responsiveness or warmth and a low level of restriction. They care about the unique needs of their child and tolerate immaturity and dysregulation. They may recognize the need for technology rules but are less likely to implement them or be consistent with consequences.

*If you answered **d** to two or more questions,* then you would be described as authoritarian. Authoritarian parents have rules that are not to be questioned. These parents often provide consistent technology rules and consequences. However, they often do not consider each child's individual desires and needs. Consequently, they achieve behavioral control, but the rules are not always internalized and generalized. They try to instill their family's values and expectations about technology by decree and not through discussion. Permissive and authoritarian styles reflect the two ends of the healthy continuum for parental warmth and control.

*Two or more **c** answers reflect an authoritative style.* Authoritative parenting is the most commonly reported style and the style most closely associated with building online resilience and digital citizenship. Here is an example of a teenage girl describing her authoritative parents.

> "My mom won't buy me the new iPhone yet. She says that my current iPhone is just fine and that I should question who my friends are if they judge me on the model of my phone. I am allowed to watch TV and post on Instagram during the week, but I have to do all of my homework first and show it to my parents before I am allowed to get on the Internet or watch videos on Hulu. My mom insists on following me on Instagram and friending me on Facebook. It is a bit weird, but she helped me manage this bullying thing that I got involved in. She made me write an apology letter and forced me to call the girl. It actually turned out okay, and I am much more careful online now.
>
> "I am allowed to go out with my friends, but I have an 11:00 P.M. curfew and have to text my mom when I change locations. She has to talk to the mother of where I am spending the night, which is totally annoying, and overkill. I had a boyfriend, but he was acting like a jerk. I broke up with him, and my mom was pretty cool about the whole thing and said that I used good judgment and might be ready for an iPhone upgrade at Christmas."

Authoritative parents strike a balance between warmth and control. They demand adherence to a code of conduct, but consequences for violations are more supportive and less punitive. They do see their children as individuals and accommodate their needs but expect their children to be socially responsible as well. Authoritative parenting has been associated with positive outcomes among adolescents in psychological and cognitive development, mental health, self-esteem, academic performance, self-reliance, and greater socialization.[5]

Permissive and authoritarian parents need to recognize the digital pitfalls in their parenting approach. In an effort to support and promote independence, a permissive parent stands the risk of not setting the expectations and guidelines needed for healthy development. Authoritarian parents manage and monitor well but stand the risk that their children will not be prepared to manage technology on their own. A balance between warmth and control leads to authoritative parenting. I have modified a diagram from Martin Valcke's study on Internet parenting style to give you a visual of the interaction between parenting styles— see below. Authoritative parents are best positioned to promote online resilience and subsequent digital citizenship.

> Authoritative parents are best positioned to promote online resilience.

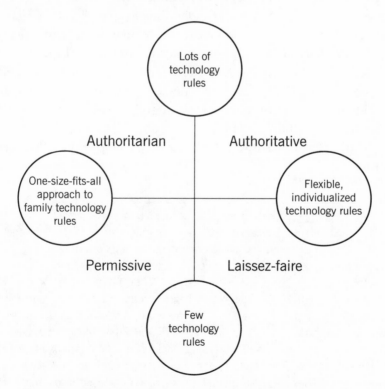

Parenting styles and Internet control. Based on Valcke et al.[6]

Candidly Assess Your Family's Technology Diet

Usage, usage, usage. The millions of statistics about digital technology generally relate to usage. Permissive and laissez-faire parents allow more use of technology. Authoritarian parents allow less. But what else drives the quantity and content of technology usage within an individual family?

There is a general notion that children drive the consumption and type of media use in a family, but how could babies and young children create the media environment in their homes? The answer is that they don't. In 2013, the Northwestern Center on Media and Development published an impressive study on parenting in the age of digital technology. They surveyed 2,300 parents of children from birth to 8 years of age. They also conducted several focus groups in California and Illinois. This study is so interesting because it is one of the first to look at younger children. In this book, I divide the statistics on usage into two groups: usage by children 8 years of age and under, and by those 9 years and over. The reason is pretty simple: Kids 8 and under often use technology with their parents and are more likely and willing to play educational games and apps. At age 9 or 10, children become literate, social, and independent. There is less media co-engagement, and the conflict begins.

The researchers at Northwestern found that parents of young children were creating different types of media environments. The study identified three different parenting styles: media-centric, media-moderate, and media-light families.[7]

Reading the descriptions below, which group do you think you fall into?

Media-centric parents: This group accounted for 39% of the participating parents. These parents love using media and spend an average of 11 hours per day on it, including more than 4 hours a day of watching TV, 3½ hours per day using the home computer, and 2 hours on their smartphones. These parents tend to keep the TV on at home most of the time even if no one is watching. Nearly half (44%) have TVs in their children's bedrooms. These parents use TV and media to connect with their kids. Although they do watch TV with their children, more than 80% of these parents report that they use TV to occupy their child when they need to make dinner or do chores. Their children spend on average 4½ hours per day on screen media. These children spend 3 hours more per day on media than children of "media-light" parents.

Media-moderate: This was the largest group, accounting for 45% of parents surveyed. These parents spend approximately 4½ hours on screen media at home. The parents play limited video games. While they like watching TV, they are less likely to list watching TV and movies as a favorite family activity. They tend to prioritize doing things as a family outside more than the media-centric families. Children in media-moderate families spend approximately 3 hours per day with screen media.

Media-light: Only 16% of families were classified as media-light. These parents spend fewer than 2 hours per day with screen media. They are much less likely to put TVs in their children's bedrooms. They are less likely to report TV and movies as a fun family activity and less likely to use TV and media to occupy their kids. Children in media-light families spend on average 1 hour, 35 minutes a day on screen media.

It is the parents' relationship with and consumption of digital technology that shapes their children's usage in the home. Parents use technology with younger children in a way that is cooperative, creative, and moderate. Technology is not a point of conflict in families with young children. Parents jointly participate in young children's media experience. They may enjoy watching a show or playing a game together, but they also prioritize and value the time they spend with their children offline.

The statistics look quite different for 8- to 18-year-olds. The Kaiser Foundation has tracked media use since 1999. In 2009, they surveyed 2,000 kids and had 700 kids keep detailed media diaries. They found that the average 8- to 18-year-old spent 7¾ hours per day using digital technology and 10¾ hours if you count using multiple devices at one time.[8] Daily use totaling 10¾ hours is mind-boggling, but what is more shocking is the increase in national usage in the 5 years from 2004 to 2009.

By 2009 kids were spending 2¼ hours more time on digital technology than they did in 2004:

- 47-minute increase in music/audio.
- 38-minute increase in TV.
- 27-minute increase in computer use.
- 24-minute increase in video games.
- No change in movies or print.

At this rate, by 2019 kids will be spending over 15 hours per day on digital media! There would be no time left to eat, sleep, or see real people. You may be reading these stats and saying there is no way your children consume that much media.

Are you sure?

I am challenging you to find out how much media you and your children really use. If you visited a nutritionist to lose weight, you would be told that you need to understand and track your eating habits before going on a diet. As with eating, technology use is best in moderation; as with counting calories, it's hard to be honest about how much time you spend on technology. Here are some pointers to keep yourself honest:

Try to keep a media diary for each member of your family for 3 days. If this exercise sounds overwhelming, then monitor each family member individually. It would be best if your children who are older than 8 years kept their own diary. I have not yet found the perfect media diary app for tracking multiple people over multiple online and offline devices. RescueTime monitors the details of Internet usages and sends you weekly graphs. TimeRabbit measures how much time you lose down the proverbial "rabbit hole" while on social media. I am not recommending that you use the parental monitoring programs for this purpose, but there is a variety of tracking software out there. Right now, we are simply doing a 3-day experiment to document how much time is spent each day on

- TV: real time, delayed, and Web-based
- Computer/tablet: online and offline activities (include homework, but star it)
- Phone: includes voice calls, texts, games, and surfing
- Gaming consoles: handheld and stationary

While all TV time should be included, I would not include music at this time unless your family is listening to music while surfing the Internet or playing a game. "Multitasking" counts more than single-tasking. If possible, highlight or underline when multitasking occurs. We are not trying to sweat the details. We want a general idea of how much time each member of your family spends with technology.

Here are my suggestions for keeping an accurate record:

■ Track hourly (not daily or weekly). If you can't do 3 days in a row, then pick a few days in a week. Be sure to include a weekend day and a weekday.

■ Send yourself a text or put a note in your calendar each time you use technology. You can also keep a paper notebook with you.

■ Consider sending text reminders to older members of your family throughout the day to remind them.

■ If you are concerned that your teenager won't be reliable, then have her send you a text message with each usage so you can track it.

■ If needed, you can look at phone usage data or utilize Rescue-Time for online activities.

■ **Be honest.**

After collecting the data, you can take an honest look at how your family uses technology. Look for problematic patterns such as late-night Internet use or extended texting during homework time. Learning how to "shut down" at night is challenging, and you may choose to get more involved in the sleep-time ritual or to turn off the Internet in your home at a certain time. In Chapter 11, I examine problematic Internet usage and help you determine whether your child is at risk. For now, we are trying to get an understanding of your family's digital habitat.

The results of your media diaries might surprise you. Usually, parents are more surprised about their usage and patterns than those of their children. Children learn by example. We all know that if Mom and Dad are texting and checking Facebook throughout dinner, then it is hardly shocking that the kids will follow suit. One of the tricks of the child psychiatry trade is knowng that parents' behavior heavily influences children's behavior, especially when kids are 12 and younger. It is quite common, for example, for an anxious 8-year-old to be referred to me. No one understands why this youngster is so anxious. I meet the parents, and it is obvious that one or both of them are extremely anxious. I will tell the parents that we need some extra parenting sessions before I meet extensively with the child. I will try to address the parents' anxiety. Sometimes I will refer the parents for their own treatment. Presto! The child's anxiety gets better. The same is true for bad media habits.

THE SECRET TO SUCCESSFUL DIGITAL PARENTING

At this point, you hopefully can accurately decorate your family's digital habitat. You can decorate the master bedroom (parents' use), the children's bedroom (children's use), the basement (children's hidden and unrecognized usage), and where it all comes together in the family room (family's approach to technology in general). The goal is to strive for authoritative parenting that combines both parental warmth and parental control. Your technology relationship and patterns will drive how and when your children use digital technology. If you are able to embrace innovation and co-engage with your child, you are likely to cultivate both online resilience and digital citizenship.

Your family's digital habitat will provide the soil for resilience and citizenship to bloom. It is your family's ongoing dialogue about digital technology that will provide the water and sunlight that your children need to prepare them for the challenges of the digital era. Your fears and ambivalences will be betrayed in these dialogues. It is essential to recognize your own concerns, but not to transmit them. Of course, you want to protect your children from the risks and pitfalls of technology. The goal is to empower your children to be critical consumers and not helpless victims. For instance, talking about TV shows and commercials can help them distinguish fantasy from reality, confront stereotypes, and lessen the effects of violence. Using the Internet together can help your children develop the subtle skills needed to ignore a mean comment or choose a positive social media site or game.

Hopefully, this chapter has helped you understand your parental identity and the context in which you function as a parent. It should be obvious by now that you must be honest and self-reflective in order to cultivate the resilience your children need to grow up in the digital era. In the last chapter of this book, you'll have a chance to create your own family technology plan based on your understanding of your family culture, in addition to everything you'll learn in the rest of this book about how digital technology can be used as a tool to support your child's growth into a resilient digital citizen.

Everything that follows in *Screen-Smart Parenting* is based on a developmental model of digital parenting. Most thoughtful approaches to parenting take into account the physical, cognitive, social, and emotional components of child development, and parenting in the digital world should be no exception.

Your children will inevitably achieve digital milestones like getting a phone, joining a social media site, or e-mailing homework to a teacher. Like developmental milestones, such

> Digital milestones come whether you are ready or not.

as walking and talking, they come whether you are ready or not. The difference with digital milestones is that parents have some say in when and how they unfold. I promise you that they *will* unfold eventually, so it is better to develop a plan and not leave it to chance and cyberspace.

2 Digital Milestones

The Facts Behind How Technology Affects Your Child's Development

As with every parenting challenge, technology does not come all at once. You don't have to worry about toilet training and sex education at the same time. This is also true for technology. Your child will learn to navigate your smartphone before you have to worry about her sexy Facebook profile picture. To help our children manage technology as they grow, we need to look at digital technology as a series of developmental or digital milestones. We need to understand each stage of our child's development and figure out which component of technology needs to be addressed then—what the child is ready for, what might be risky or otherwise age inappropriate, and, perhaps most important of all, how digital media can contribute to healthy development.

In general, a progression of exposure seems to develop. Exposure begins with TV and music. It moves to simple interactive apps and games that don't require literacy. Educational shows and games are the mainstay in the toddler and preschool years, but that changes quickly. The quality of the television and the games changes by the early school years. The educational quality of most television seems to disappear by first or second grade. With exposure to other kids in later elementary school comes the introduction of video games that are less explicitly educational. The television watching leaves the domains of PBS and Nickelodeon and enters the Disney dramas and the Cartoon Network shoot-'em-up/superhero themes. The way in which we use games and TV changes with age and time.

The big explosion in usage comes in the dreaded middle school years. Technology usage actually peaks at this time. Kids are playing video games, and socializing online begins in earnest. Most kids are given phones in middle school, and they begin to text and group chat. They will join Instagram or Snapchat. The risks for cyberbullying and hypertexting emerge in the middle school years. Social media takes on its full force toward the end of middle school and the beginning of high school. Parents begin to lose control over their child's digital footprint by the end of middle school. Therefore, our goal is to take a thoughtful approach, with rules, guidelines, and open communication in place before our children enter high school.

Knowing your family culture and technology diet is step one—consider reading Chapter 1 if you haven't already done so. Step two is understanding the developmental goals for your children—that's the subject of this chapter, and it will give you an idea of where technology fits in. Then you need to get a clear picture of the landscape—what's out there, how it all fits together. Chapters 3 and 4 help you to become fluent in the digital landscape and the primary parenting debates. By the end of the book, you will be able to draft a family technology plan. It all starts with understanding and implementing a developmental model for digital parenting.

THE EFFECT OF DIGITAL TECHNOLOGY ON YOUR CHILD'S DEVELOPMENT

As a parent, it is your job to steer your kids and teenagers in the direction of healthy development versus unhealthy. So, as you craft your approach to digital technology, you need to focus on development in the same way you do when making decisions about your child's education, nutritional choices, and physical activity.

Pediatricians and child psychiatrists tend to break growth up broadly into physical, cognitive, and social/emotional development. In the world of pediatrics, we take a multifaceted approach to your child. We care about height and weight, but that is only the beginning. Pediatricians also carefully consider cognitive, social, and emotional growth. Digital technology in all of its forms affects the daily experiences of children today and thus plays a huge role in development.

There are many different theories of child development, and all of them shed some light on how technology may affect children as they mature. For example, as I reviewed the multiple theories of child's social development that I studied in school, I was struck by the fact that most of them are relevant to the world of digital media. One goal of social and emotional development is the formation of a secure sense of self. John Bowlby, known for his attachment theory, believed that early relationships with parents and caregivers shaped relationships into adulthood. Attachment theorists might ask how television and computers can interfere with or replace relationships between babies and their parents. We know that background television interferes with the volume and quality of parent–child interactions. On the other hand, watching *Sesame Street* with your child could provide an enriching social interaction. And think about a preschool- or school-age child who is physically separated from a parent—Skype or FaceTime could provide a way to connect with that parent. Skyping should never replace real interaction, but could it be better than phones or letters in maintaining important relationships? Attachment theory is a useful tool when trying to regulate how much digital technology will creep into your baby and toddler's life. In Part II of the book, I break down the goals of social and emotional development by age to help us determine the appropriate time and age for each piece of technology.

Another example of theory relevant to digital tech decisions is Lev Vygotsky's sociocultural theory, which includes a concept called the zone of proximal development, defined as the place where a person does not have the skills or knowledge to understand or perform a task on his own but is capable of learning it with help or guidance. Taking this zone into account can inform a lot of your decisions about your child's use of digital technology. The zone is a tricky place in cyberspace. I have found, in fact, that this is precisely where kids get into trouble, because they don't have the help or guidance of wise grown-ups, like you. Younger children get frustrated when they can't understand a game or navigate a site. However, they can feel very powerful and accomplished when an adult reads the instructions or shows them how to safely access the information they are looking for. I find that younger children often don't have the cognitive skills for the games or sites that they are utilizing. Adolescents have the technical savvy needed for cyberspace but often sit in the zone of proximal development when it comes to navigating tricky social situations on social media sites.

Speaking of cognitive skills, cognition encompasses mental processes such as attention, perception, comprehension, memory, and problem solving. Cognitive development refers to changes in cognition over time. There are multiple theories of cognitive development, all of which incorporate the biological or neurological maturation that comes with life experience to create an individual who can function in a particular environment.

Cognitive development and brain development are closely related. Dr. Genevieve Johnson, an educational psychologist who studies Internet technology and human learning, explains that as your brain matures, your neuronal connections become more complex, and thus more complex cognitive processing evolves. However, the architecture of the brain is heavily dependent on your life experiences, which neuroscientists have termed "environmental stimuli." These experiences are interpreted by your brain as a pattern of neurological activity. During childhood, when brain development is highly sensitive, such activity shapes the formation of your cognitive processes. Basically, children's brain functioning is modified by patterns of cognitive demands, which hopefully result in the cognitive ability to function in a grown-up world.[1] The world of digital technology adds an entire sphere of environmental stimuli that will shape the brains of our children. For example, video games can enhance visual–spatial skills. When children are exposed to multiple and frequent video game stimuli, their neuronal pathways will adapt and visual–spatial skills will improve. Adults complain and resist the transition from paper books to e-readers. Young children, who are digital natives, easily transition between paper and screen and rarely make a distinction. There is no way to avoid the fact that digital technology is changing our brains and shaping cognitive development.

As a final example, Erik Erikson's theory of psychosocial development provides the broadest framework with which to interweave our approach to digital technology. Erikson developed a psychosocial stage theory that focused on the development of an ego identity. Ego identity is a conscious sense of self and is based on life experiences and social interactions. Each stage, according to Erikson, requires the child or adult to gain mastery over what can be viewed as a developmental crisis. Competence at each stage allows the ego identity to gain strength. Obviously we want digital technology to help kids and young adults gain competence, not feel inadequate. At stage 3, which applies to preschool-age kids, Erikson says the goal is to enable children to gain power and control by directing play and social interaction (through overcoming the crisis of initiation vs. guilt, which isn't really relevant to this discussion). Digital media can assist children as they develop more complicated play. Online, they can take more initiative in cultivating social connections. Similarly, Erikson's fifth stage (at which the crisis is autonomy vs. shame and doubt), which applies to adolescence, requires the teenager to develop a stronger sense of self and independence. Adolescents can hide in cyberspace and lose themselves in video games, or they can find like-minded friends and develop their identities through online connections.

> Understanding what children will encounter in the digital world at different stages of their growth is critical to your decision making.

Basically, digital media is a cultural tool that influences our cognition (the way we think). It is also an environmental stimulus that shapes our brain architecture. We learn by responding to patterns in our environment. Kids experience multiple and competing cues from TV and computers that influence their behavior and subsequently the development of their brain.[2] In the early years of computers, there was much fear and pessimism about the long-term impact of TV, computers, and social media on children. Over time, it has become clear that digital technology has great benefits to kids when used in moderation and safely. Let's look at what we know about the physical, cognitive, and emotional effect on development.

> 📶 This chapter gives you the bullet points about the research on development in digital media. Most of the research is cross-sectional and correlational, not causal. This means that there are strong associations but exact causes are not clear. Studies that try to prove cause and effect must have a control group and must be longitudinal, which means followed over time.

PHYSICAL DEVELOPMENT

Jake is an 11-year-old sixth grader. He comes home from school and sits in his room and watches TV. He plays World of Warcraft, which he seems to enjoy. Bedtime is a battle, and he stays up late playing games or watching TV. He quit the soccer team because he said he was too tired for the practices. He seems to be gaining weight, and his aunt suffers from diabetes. His grades are OK, but the teachers think he is working below his potential. He has friends who play World of Warcraft and Minecraft with him, but he doesn't see them in person very often.

Is Jake at risk for physical effects of digital technology? Yes. There is much publicity about the link between digital media and health. Most of the currently available research on the physical effects is based on TV and traditional video games. There is growing research on Internet use and social media, but health effects are unclear. There is very limited research on smartphone and tablet use, although I anticipate an explosion in this area in the next few years.

In excess, digital media can lead to obesity, metabolic abnormalities, and sleep disturbances. Digital technology does not *cause* any of these challenging problems. And not all technology is created equal when it comes to physical effects. However, there are some associations that are worth looking at as you develop your own media rules and opinions.

Is Digital Technology Making Us Fat?

We have an epidemic of childhood obesity in our country. The amount of TV and whether the TV is in your child's bedroom are both correlated with increased risk for obesity. The biggest culprit is television and video, which can be watched on an old-fashioned television set or streamed onto a computer, tablet, or smartphone. Most research is done on traditional television viewing.

There is debate over the mechanisms by which technology use leads to obesity, but what is clear is that excess screen time—defined as exceeding the American Academy of Pediatrics (AAP) recommendations of 2 hours per day (see Chapter 6)—and having a TV in the bedroom are linked to obesity.

The AAP policy on media, published in 2011, highlights a fascinating study done in Britain over a period of 30 years. It found that the

The presence of a TV in the bedroom makes things much worse.

higher the mean daily hours of TV viewed on weekends, the higher the body mass index (BMI) at age 30. For each additional hour of TV watched on weekends at age 5, the risk of adult obesity increased by 7%.[3] In a 2005 study of 8,000 Scottish children, researchers found that children who viewed more than 8 hours of TV per week (1.1 hours per day) at age 3 had an increased risk of obesity at age 7.[4]

Television viewing increases 1–2 hours per day when TV is watched in the bedroom. The risk of being overweight increases by 31%, and the

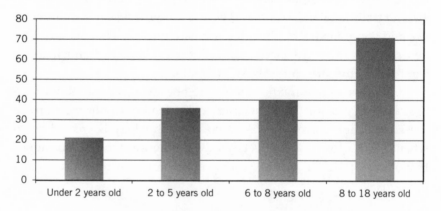

Percentage of children with TV in their bedrooms.
Data from Rideout et al. and Wartella et al.[5]

likelihood of smoking doubles.[6] A study of 2,343 children ages 9–12 years of age revealed that having a bedroom TV set was a significant risk factor for obesity independent of physical activity.[7] Teenagers with a TV in their bedroom:

- Spent more time watching TV
- Spent less time being physically active
- Ate fewer family meals
- Consumed more sweetened beverages
- Ate fewer vegetables[8]

Metabolic abnormalities that are often associated with obesity are also sometimes associated with digital technology; see the box on page 36.

When I was growing up, we played outside and didn't sit in front of screens all day. Is this change the reason kids are fat today?

Digital technology has a way of interrupting the delicate balance between caloric intake and energy expended. The evidence that digital technology replaces physical activity is not convincing, however. What is convincing is that increasing physical activity, decreasing screen time, and improving nutritional practices prevents the onset of obesity.

Some TV and video games are better than others in promoting physical versus sedentary behavior. The Wii and other interactive video game systems are my video games of choice. In a study of preteens playing Dance Dance Revolution and Nintendo's Wii Sports, the researchers found that energy expenditure was equivalent to moderate-intensity walking.[9] Wii and Xbox are TV console games that often require players to dance and jump around. Sometimes you even jump around with a friend who is physically in the same room. These games can promote human interaction and competition. In some cases TV and video games are replacing old-fashioned high-calorie-burning games, but not usually.

> The goal is to be an active, not sedentary, family and to choose good video games and television shows for your child's age and interests and use them in moderation.

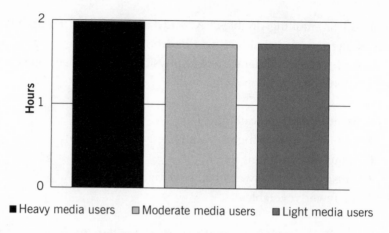

Time spent in physical activity. Adapted with permission from Rideout et al. and Wartella et al.[10]

Does technology lead to obesity by encouraging unhealthy eating habits?

Studies have shown that exposure to junk food advertising has an impact on children's food beliefs and preferences.[11] More than 80% of advertisements in children's programming are for fast foods or snacks.[12] For each hour that a child watches TV, she sees an estimated 11 food advertisements,[13] adding up to 4,400 to 7,600 ads per year according to one study—and fewer than 165 ads that promote fitness or good nutrition.[14] In one study I found very compelling, researchers found that children showed a strong preference for branded versus unbranded

Metabolic Abnormalities

There are now studies that show a correlation between heavy television viewing and hypercholesterolemia (high cholesterol), hypertension (high blood pressure), and increased prevalence of asthma.

Recent studies have also found a strong association, but not cause, between time spent watching TV and blood glucose levels in young people with type 2 diabetes, insulin resistance, and metabolic syndrome.

foods of the same type when presented with both.[15] What can you do to decrease the bombardment of ads? You can record shows (including movies, also filled with junk food references and visuals) versus watching them in real time or on demand. You can talk to your kids about the ads and point out what is going on.

> You may ultimately lose the battle to McDonald's and Cocoa Puffs, but you can help your children become more educated consumers.

My teenager refuses to shut down the computer at night. Is there a relationship to sleep and obesity?

Who hasn't stayed up too late watching a movie, texting a friend, bidding on eBay, or playing a game? However, there is evidence to support the idea that decreased sleep can lead to obesity. The mechanism may be that fatigue leads to greater sedentary behavior, which is a risk factor for obesity. It is also possible that people who are awake and sedentary may have the time and opportunity to eat more. Lastly, there is some research showing that decreased sleep may affect your neuroendocrine system and inhibit satiety (your ability to feel full).

> Do not despair. Parents can prevent their children from becoming obese and losing sleep due to digital technology.

Who Needs Sleep Anyway?

Sleep might provide us with the pathway to understanding the problematic effects of digital technology. It may be that media use results in less sleep and sleep deprivation results in myriad problems such as obesity, memory loss, and anxiety. As parents, we expend a great deal of sweat and tears managing our children's sleep habits. Parents chart sleep patterns in infants and organize their entire lives around toddlers' nap routines. In my experience, the highest level of parent–child conflict with elementary school children is around bedtime. All of this concern and drama is for good reason. Our children need to sleep. Sleep is

> Children who don't sleep are more likely to be obese, have attention problems, show irritability, and even have aggressive outbursts and temper tantrums.

restorative for the synapses and cognitive processes in our brain. Growth hormone is secreted at higher levels at night.

As a physician and a mother, I know that my children and patients need sleep. If your children are getting too little sleep, it may be affecting their development. You don't need to be a physician or neuroscientist to figure out how decreased sleep might affect development. Lack of sleep is directly related to attention problems, irritability, cognitive impairment, and obesity. That list just scratches the surface. But what *is* enough sleep? See the box below.

 ### How Much Sleep Is Enough?

Researchers at the University of South Australia looked at 300 sleep studies dating from 1897 to 2009 and found 32 sets of sleep recommendations. Most of these studies, and conventional wisdom, say that kids don't get enough sleep. This is not surprising considering that recommended sleep exceeded actual sleep in 83% of the studies. What is more shocking is that sleep recommendations are founded not on evidence-based research but on consensus—even though authors over the past century have acknowledged the lack of evidence to support their guidelines.

The truth is that kids *have* been losing sleep over the years:

- For the last 100 years, kids have been getting approximately 0.73 minutes less sleep every year.
- Children and adolescents slept 37 minutes less per night than published recommendations.[16]

It is not surprising that parents worry how their children will manage "modern times" and try to protect them with extra sleep. Ironically, we've seen a slow decline not only in actual sleep over time but also in recommendations for sleep. Recommendations for sleep dropped 70 minutes over the 20th century. The general recommendation is now 11 hours for toddlers, 10 hours ± 1 hour for school-age children, and 8 hours ± 1 hour for teenagers. The bottom line is that there is a good chance that your children are not getting enough sleep. Your children's irritable and disruptive behavior may be the first tipoff that they need more sleep.

Is technology depriving us of our sleep?

Every generation feels that the demands of technology are taxing and draining to their children. In 1905, Crichton Browne wrote, "this is a sleepless age more and more, we are turning night into day." He blamed the trolleys and streetlights; now we blame Facebook and You-Tube. There are three ways to understand how technology affects children's sleep:

1. Technology displaces sleep time (displacement hypothesis).
2. Technology causes increased emotional, cognitive, or physical stimulation, which disrupts sleep (content hypothesis).
3. Bright light exposure disrupts circadian rhythm.[17]

■ **Media replaces sleep.** The displacement hypothesis theorizes that digital technology displaces time for sleep or physical activity. In 2008, researchers found that children who spend more than 1 hour per day on TV and the Internet spend 7–10 minutes less playing, sleeping, reading, and studying.[18] However, it is more complicated than merely media replacing sleep.

■ **Computer lighting affects circadian rhythm.** Technology may not only replace sleep but actually make sleep more difficult. Melatonin is a hormone secreted by the pituitary gland for the purpose of regulating our sleep–wake cycle. It is sensitive to light and is secreted at higher levels when it gets dark at night. It has been found that exposure to a computer or iPad at maximal brightness for 2 hours can inhibit melatonin release. It is the blue light in the computers and iPads that is the worst culprit. Our sleep–wake cycle is most sensitive to lighting in the blue range. Humans are programmed to wake up to the white and blue light of sunrise. E-readers such as the Nook and Kindle have addressed this problem with their e-paper technology. E-paper technology simulates a real book. It has the look of ink. It is black and white and reflects ambient light in a room like a real paper book. Exposure to blue light in the morning can improve wakefulness and address seasonal affective disorder.[19] However, it is recommended that blue-light devices be turned off prior to sleep and not used in bed.

■ **Nighttime technology use is overstimulating.** Surfing the Internet and playing games at night has been found to increase the amount of time it takes to fall asleep and decrease the total sleep time. It delays or replaces sleep, but it is more complicated than simply displacement. The content of the technology may directly or indirectly impact the quantity and quality of sleep. Violent video games may be more disruptive of sleep than nonviolent ones even if kids are accustomed to playing more violent games. Playing violent video games increases the rate of arousal, decreases time sleeping, and can lead to poor quality of sleep.[20] A study looking at toddlers, media, and sleep found that bedtime media of all kinds and daytime media with more adult or violent themes were likely to disrupt sleep in children ages 3–5 years. However, daytime age-appropriate television did not impact the quantity or quality of sleep. Nighttime use of electronic devices has been linked to poor sleep, excess body weight, and lower physical activity.[21]

Violent content and physically and emotionally stimulating content are more problematic than passive and emotionally neutral content at night. The research and common sense tell us that digital technology disrupts sleep and needs to be minimized and managed in the evening.

COGNITIVE DEVELOPMENT

Lev Vygotsky said that human cognition creates tools (e.g., printing press, telegraph) and then in turn is created by those tools. Genevieve Johnson has taken this a step further: "The Internet is the most sophisticated tool that humans have thus far created and, as such, it may ultimately have greater cognitive impact than any previous cultural tool."[22]

> Interactive digital technology used in moderation is overwhelmingly positive in cultivating and fine-tuning your children's intelligence and education.

The impact of digital media on cognitive development is very important since cognitive development is the cornerstone of overall development. Unfortunately, most of us grown-ups are very uncomfortable with the changing cognitive demands of the digital era—it really is uncharted territory. To complicate matters, *most of the research is inconsistent and contradictory,* particularly that on the cognitive impact of digital technology on very young children. The cognitive implications for school-age children and teenagers are easier to interpret. Digital technology can be an incredible learning tool to cultivate cognitive processes that are critical to living in the 21st century, but it is important to differentiate the different genres of technology when trying to determine what makes you smarter and what makes you dumber. The big cognitive concerns are language, attention, and school performance.

Cognitive Development and Very Young Children

Technology for young children (0–5 years) is changing daily. I have three children, who are currently 5, 7, and 9 years old. When my 9-year-old was 5, he watched DVDs on a portable DVD player and played simple games on a Leapster (a simple handheld gaming device for children ages 4–10 years). My 5-year-old daughter does not own or know how to use a Leapster or portable DVD player. She downloads Bob the Builder from the App Store on our iPad and is learning to read the Bob books on the Kindle and Raz-Kids reader app. She plays Grandma's Kitchen and horrible Barbie games on my iPhone and listens to music on her brother's iPad mini. For her, it is all touch screen and interactive; nothing is passive, and very little requires real literacy. What a revolution in 4 years!

Most of our brain development is set by age 5; in fact most of it happens in the first 2 years of life. The brain grows from about 12 ounces at birth to about 35 ounces at the end of the first year. Brain weight stays about the same after age 5. However, the intricate connections called neuronal pathways develop until age 5 and then continue to reorganize. Ann DeSollar-Hale, a neuropsychologist and coauthor of *Toddlers on Technology,* very eloquently simplifies brain development.

> When explaining the brain to my patients, I like to make the analogy of walking down a path in a forest. The more times you go down the path (i.e., repetition), the larger it becomes and the easier it is to navigate. However, if you do not travel down the path, it becomes overgrown and difficult to use. These neuronal pathways are similar: the major "superhighway" connections are created early in life, during the enormous development before age

five. Pruning (weakening) begins after early development and connections or paths not used will no longer be of service. When it comes to brain development, it's a case of "use it or lose it."[23]

The "superhighway" and "tree" metaphors simplify the concept of neuroplasticity. Neuroplasticity means that our neuronal pathways are malleable and modified in response to purposeful and accidental life experiences. Don't despair if your children are older than 5 years of age. The trunk is built, but the branches and leaves can be pruned. Child and adolescent brains are "plastic" and are pruned in response to digital technology and other life experiences.

Newer research and innovation may call into question the AAP's recommendation of no screen time for children under 2 years of age (see Chapter 5). However, with the emergence of touch screens and interactive apps, babies and toddlers may be able to use iPhones and tablets to learn and grow. More than half of young children (8 years and younger) have access to an iPad, and 60% of babies (6 months to 2 years) play with laptops, computers, phones, and tablets around their homes. The emergence of smartphones and interactive tablets will undoubtedly change how we understand the cognitive impact of interactive technology.

The AAP has taken such a strong stance because it felt that early screen time could lead to language delay and attention problems. Babies and young toddlers need human interaction and real-time human voices. Human interaction is how they survive and learn. Anything that gets in the way of human interaction will lead to cognitive delays, whether it is a baby left unattended in a crib or a toddler put in front of endless hours of baby videos. In 2009, a study found that children ages 2 months to 4 years who watched excessive television had less verbal interaction and subsequent risk factors for delayed language development.[24] So the issue is not that *Sesame Street* or Baby Einstein causes language delay. Excessive TV viewing has been found to lead to less volume and quality of human interaction, which subsequently may lead to cognitive delays.

The concerns about attention are related to babies' developing brains and level of engagement. Babies and young toddlers have difficulty converting 2D images into 3D. They are more engaged by real people or something that is truly interactive. Passive TV is always passive TV, whether it is *Howdy Doody* on a large 1950s TV or *Dora the Explorer* downloaded onto an iPad mini.

I agree with the AAP recommendation for no traditional TV prior to age 2 and for less than 2 hours per day after 2 years of age. It is the smartphone and interactive tablet that hold the most promise for cognitive development in younger children. The writers of *Toddlers on Technology* make a compelling argument for how the new technology can cultivate young children's cognitive skills and ultimately their

> TV viewing is not ideally suited to keep young children engaged and to foster their attention span.

school performance. There is not enough (or basically any) research yet, because Digitods (those born after the inception of the iPhone in 2007) and smartphone/tablet technology are too new. However, there is a lot of anecdotal evidence. The educators who wrote *Toddlers on Technology* observed that preschool kids were much more interested in flash card apps than traditional flash cards regardless of how fancy they made the traditional cards. The apps were interactive and allowed the toddlers to feel in control, and they provided needed repetition without boring the adults to death. Teachers have seen young children attend to these programs in ways that they have not seen with traditional teaching tools. We may find that interactive educational technology improves attention span in toddlers and young children. It is likely that we will see significant cognitive and educational effects with the newer interactive technology.

What about School-Age Kids?

Can digital technology prepare kids for school and make them smarter?

Yes. Interactive technology used in moderation makes you smarter. It cultivates critical cognitive processes, which by definition makes you smarter. The question is whether it helps school performance. Let's start with the positives and come back to school performance.

Most of the research on cognitive development relates to young children. A review of the research by Moses found that moderate amounts of television were beneficial for reading but that the content of television matters.[25] They also found that programs that aim to promote literacy in young children did promote literacy. Once children gain basic literacy skills around ages 7–8, television has not been found to cultivate more complex comprehension and interpretation skills.

Genevieve Johnson developed a diagram to help people understand the cognitive impact of digital technology. I have modified it for our use (see below), but it gives you a nice visual of the types of cognitive skills that are related to video game, Internet, and social media use. (Television is not on the diagram because for the most part TV is not cognitively demanding and does not cultivate any cognitive skills, although some educational TV may increase kids' knowledge base and passively expose children to new experiences and social interactions.) In moderation, technology promotes multiple cognitive processes.

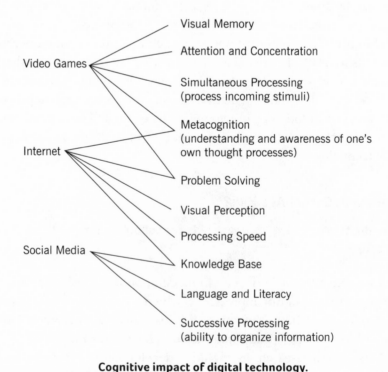

Cognitive impact of digital technology.
Adapted with permission from Johnson.[26]

What effect do video games have?

The cognitive risks and benefits of video games include:

- Playing video games increases response time performance.
- It teaches you how to process and organize a variety of competing stimuli.
- It gives kids lots of practice in visual–spatial skills.
- Children who play video games have been found to be better at rotating shapes and seeing shapes in 3D.
- Children who play video games are more likely to read instructions on their own and use trial and error to problem-solve.[27]
- Video game players have strong visual memory and are good at pattern recognition.

All of these skills are parts of our cognitive process and components of how we define intelligence. Video games may seem mindless and a waste of time to parents, but they have the ability to truly sharpen the cognitive skills of the player.

How does Internet use affect development?

Reading a website is not like reading a book. It is more interactive and requires more decision making than reading a book. The reader must employ search strategies and evaluate the credibility of a site. It forces the user to manage multiple competing stimuli like pop-ups and hypertext. It is an incredible source of information. The question is no longer "Can I find the answer to the question?" but rather how to choose and integrate multiple explanations and answers. I tried to define *encyclopedia* for my 7-year-old son. I told him that it was a group of books that held all of the answers that Google did. He looked at me like I was crazy and said that they must be very big books.

Nicholas Carr in *The Shallows* laments the fact that we read differently online. It is no longer from left to right or top to bottom. We skim and scan and search for relevant information.[28] This may be true, but researchers have found that literacy programming on TV and computer games does improve reading in younger kids. Television and the Internet may boost traditional reading skills in addition to the newer demands of the Internet. Since kids do not go to the encyclopedia any-more, they need to learn how to scan, skim, and jump around. The goal is to learn this style of reading without sacrificing the traditional thoughtful, slower style of reading.

Will digital technology bring my child's grades up or down?

School performance and cognitive development are related but not the same. Screen time that exceeds 2 hours per day, late-evening screen time, and technology in the bedroom are risk factors for poor school performance. This does not necessarily mean that the technology makes you dumber, but it might make you a worse student. There are two theories to explain poor school performance: the displacement and content hypotheses. The displacement hypothesis says that screen time displaces time for sleep and studying. The content hypothesis focuses on the content of media that has a direct effect on cognition, attention, and schoolwork. Sharif and Sargent found that both displacement and content were risk factors for poor school performance.[29] Weekday screen time (TV and video games) was a risk factor for poor school performance, but weekend screen time was not. They also found that more exposure to adult content was related to sensation seeking, rebel-liousness, and poor school performance.

The pathway between adult content and poor school performance is not clear. While technology is supposed to make us more efficient, this may not be the case with preteens and teenagers and their school-work. Multitasking and constant bombardment from multiple devices may interfere with more focused studying. Digital technology can be distracting and intrusive. It can be difficult for children to have unin-terrupted time to think, organize, and analyze. In moderation digital technology is great for your cognitive development. In excess and in the bedroom and without parental supervision and rules, it can dis-place physical activity, sleep, and social interaction.

SOCIAL AND EMOTIONAL DEVELOPMENT

Generally, social and emotional development refers to children and adolescents' ability to develop relationships, self-regulate emotions, and engage in the outside world. Children must develop a strong sense of self and an ability to express emotions in order to form meaningful relationships. While most research on cognitive development focuses on young children, the research on the social effects of digital technology focuses on tweens and teenagers. I have broken up this discussion into four sections that are relevant to digital technology:

- The science of play
- Social media and self-esteem
- Digital technology and friendship formation
- Online connectedness versus loneliness

The Science of Play

Play and exploration form the cornerstone of early identity formation. In recent years we've seen a shift back to encouraging kids to play. Nursery schools focus less on knowledge acquisition and more on play and creativity. The most elite Manhattan nursery schools pride themselves on not formally teaching reading and not drilling math facts. They offer opportunities for structured and unstructured play.

Modern interactive technology can be integrated seamlessly into early childhood education but should not replace real-life play in this age group. Sharing an iPad in nursery school fosters reciprocal play but is not substantially different from sharing crayons or toys. **The real treasure of digital technology is that it offers older kids the opportunity for imaginative play.**

> Technology offers a virtual playground to older children.

If only I had a nickel for every time a parent said to me, "When I was young we played in the backyard, and now my children are over-scheduled and playing video games inside." Most mothers who come into my office will rattle off a list of their child's activities. The self-aware parent will include a designated day for playdates so that play is scheduled and is a somewhat valued pursuit. It is wonderful when a 12-year-old boy builds a fort outside and plays cowboys with the neighborhood kids. But by middle school, kids are often too self-conscious to play even if there is an assigned time slot. Traditional console

> Only in the 21st century can you continue to play "house" or "school" into adulthood.

games, role-playing games, and the Internet in general offer a rich opportunity for play and subsequent identity development.

There are endless examples of online games that allow kids, teens, and adults opportunities to be playful and creative. Kids can create avatars or alternate identities and live out fantasy adventures. Minecraft allows kids to play with blocks and create complicated structures. In World of Warcraft, you build powerful avatars and join guilds where teammates work closely together and often communicate and meet off- and online. Second Life allows you to become a different person and live out a fantasy life. The avatars in Second Life make "life" choices and have online relationships and families. The Internet and video games can be safe places to try out different identities and fantasies.

Once again, content and timing matter in the digital era. Excessively violent games may desensitize the player to violence or lead to more aggressive behavior. Adult content sites and games may expose kids and teenagers to inappropriate content. Age-inappropriate games may be frustrating and demoralizing for younger children. Excessive game playing or Web surfing can displace sleep and real-life interaction. However, the Internet and both online and offline games can provide spaces for play and fantasy ideally suited for preadolescent and adolescent identity development.

Social Media and Self-Esteem

Ideally a solid sense of self develops in early childhood, and a more sophisticated identity evolves throughout adolescence. The aspect of "sense of self" that you need to understand when evaluating the catch-all phrase "self-esteem" is the self-conscious awareness of self—the part of you that reflects and evaluates yourself. The "earlier" research (by which I mean late 1990s and early 2000s) trended toward the idea that the Internet and social networks caused depression and loneliness. More recent research focuses on how Facebook and other social networks can lead to social connectedness, including how social media can actually cultivate sense of self by allowing user control over the identity presented and refined online.

Social media allows for **selective self-presentation.** The user has control over how his or her identity is portrayed online by choosing pictures to post, people to "friend," and music and sites to "like," "tweet," or "pin." We all have an actual and ideal self, and social media sites can trigger your "ideal self," which can ultimately lead to a more positive sense of self or self-esteem.

Gonzales and Hancock did a fascinating study that highlights how Facebook can trigger positive self-representation. They took 63 students from a university and put them in three groups: one control group, one group at individual cubicles with a mirror, and one group at individual cubicles with a computer and their Facebook profiles open. The participants were told that it was an experiment about people's attitudes about themselves after exploring the Internet, and they were asked to fill out a survey. The Facebook group scored the highest on self-esteem. Even more interesting, the group that modified their profiles during the 3-minute window had the highest self-esteem ratings. The ability to present your "ideal" self online and modify as you choose may actually boost your general sense of self and self-esteem. When used responsibly, it seems that the Internet and social networking can be powerful tools for building self-esteem and cultivating your "ideal self."

The power of self-presentation is sometimes neutralized by presentation anxiety or social media depression. In Chapter 11, I address the challenges for children and adolescents who suffer from anxiety or struggle with poor social skills, depression, and anxiety. Basically, those who suffer from poor self-esteem or social anxiety may not be as well equipped to take advantage of the tools that digital technology has to offer.

Digital Technology and Friendship Formation

> **Is social media destroying my teenager's ability to develop real relationships?**

The answer to that question 10 years ago would have been yes. Today the answer is *no*, but it depends on whom you ask. Valkenburg and Peter, two Dutch researchers, have explained that 10 years ago the Internet was a place where you connected with strangers online at the expense of your "real-life" friends. Several studies in the late 1990s showed that adolescent Internet use reduced teenagers' social connectedness and well-being.[30] Now almost all young people are online, and most of them use the Internet to initiate and strengthen their "real-life" friendships.

Researchers suggest that, because online communication stimulates self-disclosure, the Internet is good for adolescent relationships. Adolescents are more likely to disclose intimate information online than in real life. The emerging research shows a slight gender shift. Boys are more likely than girls to disclose information online that they would not disclose in person. Moderate self-disclosure enhances the quality of friendships. There is research supporting the idea that online self-disclosure is related to friendship formation and to the rating of friendships as "high quality." The Dutch researchers found that in 1 year adolescents' online disclosure resulted in higher-quality friendships. Online disclosure doesn't cause better friendships, but it contributes to what is needed for a high-quality friendship. Finally, research supports the idea that high-quality friendships promote well-being. So online communication and self-disclosure can help adolescents develop stronger online and offline friendships.

The goal of adolescence and early adulthood is to develop meaningful and intimate relationships outside of the family. Technology has certainly changed the nature of our relationships. The change has been unsettling for digital immigrants but need not be viewed as inherently problematic. Digital natives are more comfortable with cyber boyfriends and virtual relationships. They move fluidly between "virtual" and "real" friends. Most teenagers and adults prefer real interaction versus online. However, there is a role for virtual relationships, and not all relationships formed in cyberspace are created equally. It is possible for adolescents to form safe, supportive, and collaborative relationships online. The trick is not to allow them to replace or overshadow face-to-face interaction and relationships. The Internet and social network sites are invaluable new tools that can cultivate existing friendships and promote meaningful virtual relationships.

Online Connectedness versus Loneliness

Sherry Turkle, founder of the MIT Institute on Self and Technology and author of *Alone Together*, tells us that digital connections lead to an "illusion of companionship." While this view is highly publicized, it tells only half of the story. Adolescents use the Internet and social media to keep in touch, make plans, and share pictures, thoughts, and ideas. Teenagers with positive self-esteem and good technology skills find support online when they are confused about a homework assignment, sick at home, or sad about a recent breakup. Teenagers can use digital technology to maintain and cultivate real friendships. They can also make virtual friends who often share interests and skills. Virtual friends can edit poetry, correct a mistake in a teen's coding project, or become teammates in a virtual gaming adventure. Digital technology holds endless potential for initiating, maintaining, and strengthening real and virtual friendships.

The caveat is that when the Internet is put into inexperienced hands or misused, it can be detrimental to social connectedness and relationships. For example, researchers found that when college students sought excessive reassurance on Facebook, they got negative feedback. Facebook became a source of social isolation, sometimes profound, not support, and it also put them at risk for low self-esteem.[31] Adolescents and young adults with poor social skills, depression, and anxiety are more likely to inappropriately self-disclose and excessively seek reassurance online. My clinical experience and the research support the idea that adolescents with poor social and technology skills often feel much more isolated and lonely when they are online. (See Chapter 11 for ways to help your vulnerable adolescent.)

I believe that the developmental model of digital parenting is integral in helping your child capitalize on the potential of technology, instead of falling prey to the pitfalls. The Internet and social media are emerging and complicated tools that need to be taught, supervised, and introduced slowly over time since they require a degree of maturity. In the next chapter I give you a map of the digital landscape so you have a good overview of what devices, media, services, apps, and games your child will encounter and what usage looks like at various ages.

3 The Digital Landscape

What You Need to Know about the Tech Terrain

Sixteen-year-old Stacy was referred to me for low-grade depression and "not reaching her academic potential." She is an extraordinarily bright teenager who uses her intelligence as a buffer against dealing with her own feelings. Like many her age, she has learned advanced computer science and calculus, but using a calendar and doing homework efficiently remain a challenge. She explained that she was perfectly capable of running multiple computer programs while simultaneously doing her homework. I suggested that she try using the SelfControl or Self Restraint apps to protect her time. In my heavily accented Digital-ese, I explained that these apps allow you to set a timer and choose problematic websites to block. For instance, you can block Facebook and YouTube for 2 hours while doing your homework. Your Internet is fully functional, but there are fewer distractions.

Very sweetly, Stacy began to speak more slowly and loudly, the way people do when talking to someone who doesn't fully understand their language. She explained that SelfControl was not an app but rather a "Web browser extension." (It actually is an app.) She explained that such programs were useless because she had her computer configured to circumvent them with three keystrokes. I felt myself panicking. I am proficient in Digital-ese but far from fluent. I didn't have the language to have a sophisticated discussion or to counter her argument. I responded that three keystrokes might still be a good reminder to keep her off distracting sites.

My interaction with Stacy probably sounds familiar to you. It is hard to keep up with digitally fluent teenagers. When I graduated from the University of Pennsylvania in 1992, we were required to be "proficient" in a foreign language, not fluent. Today, parents must be proficient in Digital-ese so they can translate and interpret their children's digital lives. Don't fear—it is not necessary to sign up for an immersion course. You have a tutor sitting right next to you—your child. If your child is under 10, you can learn together, but don't be surprised if your child surpasses you by the second class.

When I was learning about computers in middle school, the big distinction was between software and hardware. Today we talk about different types of media platforms and their overlapping interactions. In the technology world, *platform* refers to the hardware or software that other applications are built on. Computing platforms include Windows PC and Macintosh. Mobile platforms include Android, iPhone, and Palm's webOS.[1] A social networking service is a platform for building social networks or social relations among people who share common interests or activities. Social networking is generally a Web-based service that allows individuals to create public profiles and interact with each other over the Internet. The definitions and distinctions are often blurry and overlapping. Facebook started out as a simple social networking site. It has evolved into its own media platform, since games, applications, and videos are now designed to run on Facebook.

I have broken up the current digital landscape into the following broad platforms:

- TV
- Mobile media
- Computer
- Video games
- Social networking services

Platforms are, of course, only one part of the picture. The increased speed and availability of the Internet, the emergence of mobile devices, and touch-screen technology have all contributed to the current digital landscape. The increase in the speed of the Internet and the increased accessibility of the Internet have allowed more people to participate

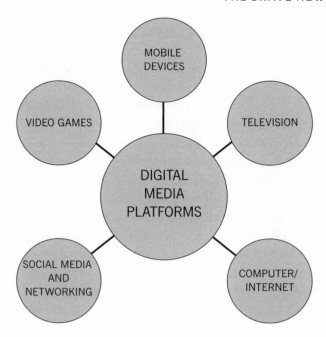

in the digital revolution. Parents need to understand the distinctions between the keyboarding, touch-screen, and no-touch interfaces. Traditionally, we use a keyboard, mouse, or joystick to navigate a computer or a game. The advent of the iPad brought a touch-screen revolution that has driven consumption, particularly among younger children who were unable to manipulate a mouse or read a keyboard. The future of technology may lie in voice-activated interaction such as the iPhone's Suri. The mobility of our devices has given us more time and opportunity to use technology. For better or worse, digital technology is ubiquitous. Our devices can be found at home and at school, in our pockets and under our pillows.

In the rest of this chapter, I outline key definitions you can use to map your child's digital landscape.

21ST-CENTURY TV

TV occupies a huge plot on the digital landscape. In fact it takes up the majority of time spent on digital technology. Children spend more time watching TV than they do in school.[2] TV has both changed and stayed the same. Families continue to watch sitcoms, reality shows, dramas, and movies. However, the way in which we view TV has evolved. The time spent watching live TV is dropping as Web-based TV takes it place. Kids increasingly watch TV on iPods, MP3 players, smartphones, tablets, and computers.

Web-based TV has become its own industry. In the early 2000s, broadband became more available and bandwidth increased, and thus "streaming" TV online became more practical. By 2009, the International Academy of Web Television had been formed, with its own Streamy Awards. Original programming is no longer confined to networks or cable TV. The most popular sites used to stream shows include YouTube, Netflix, Vimeo, Yahoo Screen, Dailymotion, and Hulu. All of these sites produce original programming and provide a

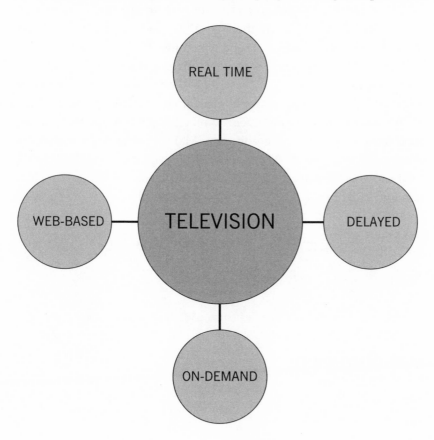

huge library of classics and recently released shows. Networks' home sites, YouTube, and other sites often offer shows for free, but everything can be streamed or downloaded for a price. Kids talk about watching "series," not shows. My patients tell me that they are halfway through the first season of *Friends* or on to the second season of *Hogan's Heroes*. They think less about 30-minute and 60-minute shows. They download series and watch one show after another. The evolution of TV runs even deeper. Very young children don't easily grasp the concept of live TV anymore. They pinch and swipe TV screens and expect that their favorite show will magically appear—and it does.

Kids see TV as a foundation for "multitasking." I will say more about the myth of multitasking in the next chapter. Most kids report that they "multitask" while watching TV. Weekly family viewing of *The Love Boat* or *Charlie's Angels* has evolved into kids watching TV on tablets while doing something else, like texting, surfing, or homework. Approximately 70% of 7th through 12th graders multitask at some point with another medium while watching TV.[3]

TV has also become more interactive. It started with voting for your favorite contestant on *American Idol* and has evolved into tweeting, posting, and voting throughout a variety of shows. Kids will watch TV together from their own bedrooms with constant chatting, instant messaging (IM), or texting going on. Many kids look up information about the characters or shows during the program. While TV viewing has become more varied and interactive, it can still lead to procrastination and sedentary behavior if viewed excessively and in the bedroom.

SOME STATISTICS ABOUT TV THAT YOU SHOULD KNOW

- Eleven- to 14-year-olds watch the greatest amount of TV, averaging about 3 hours per day.
- Black and Hispanic children watch more TV than white children across all platforms, even when controlling for age, gender, parent education, and family composition.
- Seventy percent of children have TVs in their bedrooms.
- Young children who have TVs in their bedroom spend 1 hour more watching TV each day than those who do not have a TV in their bedroom.

- Approximately 50 percent of children live in homes where the TV is left on when no one is watching it (i.e., background TV).
- Parents are more likely to set rules about what children watch (46%) than how much time they spend watching (28%).[4]

Below you'll find a list of vocabulary words and sites that parents should know.

 Modern TV Vocabulary Words

Podcasts: Digital audio or video files that can be downloaded or streamed from the Internet to a computer, portable media player, or other device.

Streaming: A method of sending data like audio and video content over a computer network so it can be watched in real time. Instead of downloading and then watching or listening, you play it while subsequent content is being sent.

Time-shifted TV: TV programming that you record and then store on a device (e.g., DVR, TiVo) or via a cable service to be watched at a later time.

Web TV: Original TV content produced specifically to be broadcast on the Internet.

YouTube: The largest video-sharing site on the Web, with 1 billion monthly visitors. Anyone can upload short videos for public or private viewing.

Netflix: A U.S. provider of TV and movie content subscriptions, available either on demand via Internet streaming or by mail-order DVDs. Its mail-order digital distribution service started in 1999 and by 2009 had 10 million subscribers. Ironically, Blockbuster declined to buy it for $50 million in 2000. Currently, it has 150 million monthly visitors. Netflix has led the way in original Web-based programming. Its *House of Cards* won the first-ever major Emmy award for a Web-based program in 2013.[5]

MOBILE MEDIA PLATFORM

It is the mobile media platform that has driven the increased consumption of digital technology. For today's kids, a cell phone is hardly ever just a phone. Cell phones are now considered mobile media delivery platforms. In fact, kids are talking on the phone less and using it for everything else more and more. Your kids will use their phones to talk, text, listen to music, read, take pictures, play games, shop, surf the Internet, and watch TV. Traditional TV viewing has dropped while watching TV on a phone or tablet has increased. The increase in video game use over the last 10 years has been mostly attributable to handheld gaming devices and games played on phones and tablets. Cell phone ownership among teens and tweens is two to three times as high as it was 10 years ago. **Currently, one-quarter of all third graders own a cell phone.** Approximately 75–85% of teenagers own a cell phone, and half of those teens own a smartphone.[6]

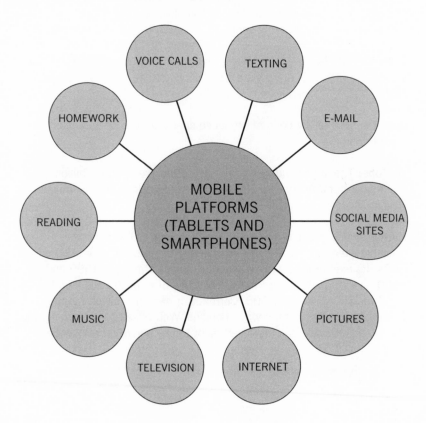

For most kids, electronic communication starts with texting and progresses to social media over time. Basically, texting starts as soon as a child owns a phone, tablet, or MP3 player and continues to ramp up throughout adolescence. Electronic communication has changed the way we communicate. I will talk more about the texting revolution, but you need to understand that texting may be the best way to communicate with your kids at times. I am not saying that texting should replace real-life interaction, but you may find it a good way to communicate and stay connected to your kids as they grow up.

> Almost all kids use the texting function on their phone more than any other function.

CELL PHONE USAGE BY TODAY'S KIDS AND TEENS

- Teens average 3,000 texts per month.
- Teens average 120 phone calls per month.
- Some teens exceed 10,000 texts per month.[7]
- An 8- to 18-year-old spends 30 minutes per day making traditional voice calls.
- An 8- to 18-year-old spends 1½ hours per day texting.
- Only 14% of teens have rules about the number of texts they can send per day.[8]

A text message is defined as an electronic message sent over a cellular network, usually from one handheld device to another. Today texts include written words, pictures, videos, memes (i.e., images that convey an idea, theme, joke, or commentary), and emoticons. Communication has become shorter and more visual. Children are able to stay in constant contact with their parents in a way that was never possible before. The constant contact has its pros and cons, which we will explore throughout the book. On the positive side, you can keep track and stay involved with your youngsters' lives in a much more seamless way. However, I see many college students and young adults who can't function or make decisions on their own because they carry their parents with them at all times via their phone. Smartphones and constant texting may infantilize young adults. The author of an article titled "A Nation of Wimps" labeled the cell phone as the "eternal umbilicus."[9] Kids should begin to learn to manage texting in middle school.

Parents have to strike a balance between constant communication and encouraging the independence and self-confidence that growing up is all about.

Parents should be able to define sexting (see Chapters 4, 9, and 10) and selfies. *Sexting* is defined as the sending of sexually explicit photographs or messages, usually between mobile phones. In August 2012, the term was officially listed in the *Merriam-Webster Collegiate*

 Mobile Device Vocabulary Words

Chat: Any kind of communication over the Internet. Traditionally, it refers to one-to-one communication through a texting application such as instant messaging.

Emoticon: A representation of facial expressions, such as :-) to express a smile, made up of various keyboard characters. Emoticons are used to convey the writer's feelings or signal the intended tone.

Emoji: Ideograms or smileys used in Japanese electronic messages that have spread beyond Japan. The icons have been standardized and are built into the new smartphones and into e-mail services such as Gmail.

Screenshot: (screen-cap/screengrab): An image created by the user (most likely on a computer or phone) to record the visible items displayed on the monitor, TV, or other visual output device.

Selfie: A photograph taken of oneself, typically with a smartphone or webcam, and uploaded to a social media site.

Sexting: The sending of sexually explicit photographs or messages via cell phone. As many as 80% of 21-year-olds have received a sext.

Snapchat: A photo messaging application where users can send photos, videos, text, and drawings to a list of designated recipients. The photos and videos sent are called "snaps." Users set the maximum time limit, from 1 to 10 seconds, that recipients can view their snaps, after which the image supposedly disappears from the recipient's device. Caveat: the recipient can take a screenshot of the image so that it sticks around. Snapchat and similar applications have become breeding grounds for sexting and cyberbullying.

Dictionary. Sexting begins on text before kids even enter the world of social media. We discuss sexting in further detail later, but you need to know the term now and how it interacts with the devices that your tweens and teens are using.

Selfie became an official word in 2013, and it has begun to define the current generation. *Selfie* is generally defined as a self-portrait photograph taken with a smartphone camera or webcam. It has become the mainstay of photo-sharing social media sites like Instagram. I talk more about these self-portraits and *Selfie,* the movie, in Chapter 10. It is important for parents to understand that selfies are more than a picture for a digital photo album. Kids use selfies to convey an idea, a thought, or a moment. Most kids don't overthink or overpose their selfies. Selfies have simply become another way of communicating in the 21st century. Some basic definitions you should know about the mobile device platform are in the box on page 60. A lexicon of texting abbreviations is below.

 Texting Abbreviations

My research assistant, Lola Seaton, age 18 at the time of this writing, compiled this short list of texting abbreviations to get you started. We could fill this entire book with a list of texting abbreviations, which continue to get shorter and more difficult to decipher.

ATM: At The Moment	ILY: I Love You
BF: BoyFriend	IMO: In My Opinion
BFF: Best Friend Forever	JK: Just Kidding
BRB: Be Right Back	K/KK: Okay
BTW: By The Way	KL: Cool
DMC: Deep Meaningful Conversation	LMAO: Laughing My Ass Off
DW: Don't Worry	LOL: Laughing Out Loud
FB: FaceBook	LUSM: Love You So Much
FBC: FaceBook Chat	LY: Love You
GF: GirlFriend	NM: Never Mind/Not Much
GTG: Got To Go	NP: No Problem
IDC: I Don't Care	OMG: Oh My God
IDK: I Don't Know	PLS/PLZ: Please

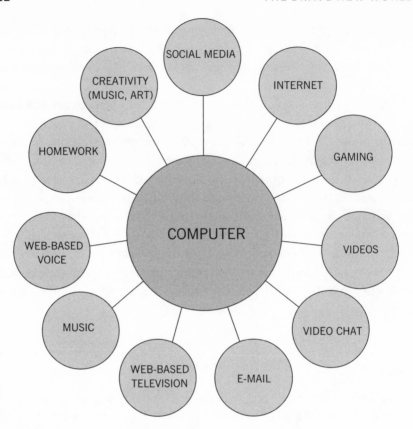

COMPUTER PLATFORM

Despite the mobile and touch-screen revolutions, children and teenagers continue to use computers for approximately 1½–2 hours per day. This does not include schoolwork or time spent watching TV and listening to music on the computer.

HOW 8- TO 18-YEAR-OLDS SPEND THEIR COMPUTER TIME (NOT INCLUDING TV, MUSIC, OR HOMEWORK)

- Social networking, 22 minutes
- Games, 17 minutes
- Video websites (e.g., YouTube), 15 minutes

- Other websites, 11 minutes
- E-mail, 5 minutes
- Graphics/photos, 4 minutes
- Reading magazines/newspapers, 2 minutes
- Anything else, 2 minutes
- Total: 1 hour, 29 minutes (1 hour, 46 minutes for 11- to 14-year-olds)[10]

Call Grandma on the Computer?

The trend in voice calling and videoconferencing is to use the computer, not the landline. The acronym is **VoIP**. VoIP stands for "voice over Internet protocol." It is also called IP telephone or Internet phone. VoIP allows you to speak or video over the Internet. It is available on most smartphones, computers, and other devices with Internet access. At this point, the audio quality is still lower than on phone lines, but it is likely that phone lines are going the way of the beeper and the

---

The Computer: Encouraging Reading and Research?

The era of reading is certainly not over, but it does seem to be shifting from paper to the computer, tablets, and smartphones. Reading on devices and computers is taking up a larger percentage of overall reading. In the last 5 years, there has been a huge shift in the type of literacy programs you can find online for young children. I believe that the Digitods (those born since the inception of the iPhone in 2007) will truly learn to read on the computer and tablets. Kids also get critical information online by reading websites and doing research. Fifteen- to 18-year-old girls (66%) are more likely to have looked up health information online than to have watched TV, listened to the radio, or posted video online.[11] I often see teenage patients who look up health information for friends or themselves online and then come into my office to verify or clarify the information. These questions frequently open up meaningful dialogue about health and sexuality. Children will increasingly use the Internet and their digital devices for reading and research. The goal is to find good educational tools and learn how to be critical consumers who value authenticity and copyright.

Walkman. Examples of VoIP are Skype, FaceTime, TeamSpeak, and Viber. You may feel that your teenager is isolated in his bedroom, but he may be FaceTiming or Skyping with school friends while also playing a video game with his "virtual friends" from around the world. The big question is not whether he is lonely but whether he is doing his homework.

VIDEO GAME PLATFORM

Video games are not the arcade games of our youth. However, I do love that Pac-Man has been revived as a cartoon superhero on the Disney channel. Video games have come a long way since the Pac-Man and Donkey Kong in the mall arcade. I have divided up gaming into five major types:

- Arcade games (think 1980s malls)
- Stationary gaming consoles
- Handheld gaming devices
- Simpler games that can be played easily on phones, tablets, and computers
- More complicated massive multiplayer games for PCs

A **video game console** is a device that allows users to play video games on a separate TV in contrast to a handheld device or traditional arcade game. The Magnavox Odyssey was the first console game in 1972, but it was Atari's video game Pong that popularized home video game consoles. Apparently there was a video game crash in the mid-1980s, and it was Nintendo Entertainment Systems that revitalized home video game consoles. Microsoft's Xbox, Sony's PlayStation, and Nintendo's Wii series are the main players right now. The 2014 leaders are the Sony PlayStation 4, the Microsoft Xbox One, and the Nintendo Wii U. These consoles are Internet connected, and kids can download games for the consoles and play with others via the Internet connection. New game consoles also offer video streaming services like Netflix or Hulu.[12]

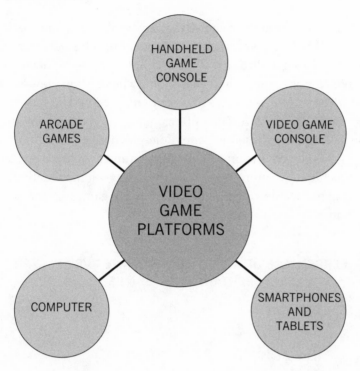

A **handheld game console** is a lightweight portable electronic device with built-in screen, speakers, and game controllers. It is smaller than a traditional stationary game console. Handheld consoles were first introduced in the late 1970s but popularized by Nintendo's Game Boy in 1989 and its signature game, Tetris. In 2004, the Game Boy was essentially replaced by Nintendo's DS series, and Sony released its PlayStation Portable device (PSP) series. In 2014, the hottest devices are Nintendo's 3DS and Sony's PS Vita (the PSP update).

Only about half of gaming takes place on video game consoles. The rest takes place on portable devices: handheld players (29%) and cell phones (23%). Video game playing peaks in the 11- to 14-year-old group. Younger kids spend more time than older kids on handheld devices like the Nintendo DS, Sony PSP, or the iPod Touch. Both boys and girls play games on portable devices, but boys spend much more time on console devices. Boys can spend an average of an hour on a console player compared to 15 minutes for girls.

There are thousands of games that can be played on mobile devices and computers. Plants vs. Zombies, Temple Run, Subway Surfers, Clash of Clans, and Angry Birds are a few examples of games that are easily downloaded onto phones and played anywhere. Many games can be played on both mobile devices and computers. Minecraft has a pocket edition and a PC edition. The options, updates, and graphics are better for the computer-based version. Role-playing games with multiple players generally have complicated graphics and are played on computers. As technology improves and everything goes mobile, there is an increasing number of role-playing and fantasy games for the Android and iPhones.

PERCENTAGE OF KIDS 8–18 WHO HAVE EVER PLAYED CERTAIN VIDEO GAMES

- Guitar Hero, 71%
- Super Mario, 65%
- Wii Play/Sports, 64%
- Grand Theft Auto, 56%
- Halo, 47%
- Madden NFL, 47%

Video Game Genres

Surprisingly, there is no real consensus on genres of video games. Still, it's helpful to know some general categories.[13] Showing interest in your child's games will allow you to better understand his digital world.

Action Games

The action genre is the largest category of games and is composed of a multitude of subgenres. Basically, action games involve physical challenges, hand–eye coordination, and reaction time. The three most important types are the fighter games, the shooter games, and the platform games. In an action game, the player typically controls the

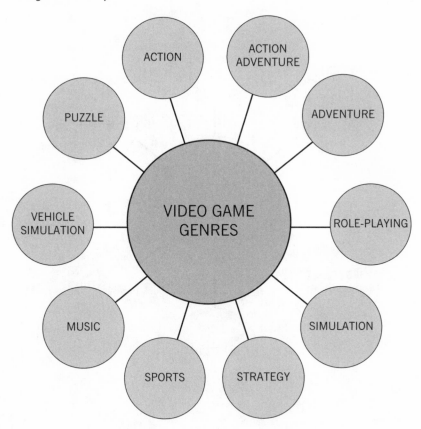

protagonist. The protagonist (called an avatar) must navigate a level, collect objects, avoid obstacles, and battle enemies. Sometimes the avatar will win by finishing levels or defeating enemies. Some games are unwinnable and the goal is to amass as many points/coins as possible. Here are some examples:

- **Basic ball and paddle games** like the classic Pong.
- **Fighting games:** Fighting between two characters where one is computer controlled (e.g., Street Fighter, Mortal Kombat).
- **Platform games:** These games involve traveling between platforms by jumping. Characters often climb ladders and ledges. Donkey Kong was one of the first examples. Nintendo's Super Mario series is one of the most successful and enduring series of

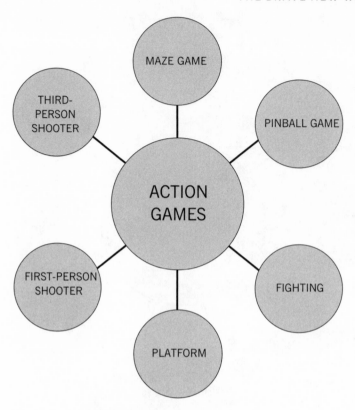

all time. The platform genre was the most popular style of game at the end of the 20th century.

- **Shooter games:**
  - ☐ First-person shooter (FPS): The emphasis is on shooting and combat from the perspective of a character (e.g., Halo and Call of Duty).
  - ☐ Third-person shooter: These games involve shooting and combat where the character/player is seen from a distance— wider camera angle (e.g., Resident Evil, Gears of War).

Other Game Genres

- **Adventure:** These were some of the earliest games created. They do not require fast reflexes or reaction time. They require a player to solve a variety of puzzles by interacting with people or the environment. These games built the foundation for the more elaborate role-playing games. Myst is an example of an influential adventure game from the 1990s.

- **Simulation:** This is a broad category of games generally designed to simulate real events or fictional reality. Players may build, expand, or manage a fictional community. Minecraft is an example of a construction and management simulation game. SimCity is an example of a city-building game.
- **Music genre:** Players interact with music and try to follow along with beats or rhythms. They may use a dance pad or a replica of an instrument. Music games have been a foundation for exergaming and have made video games more socially interactive. Popular games include Dance Dance Revolution and Guitar Hero.
- **Sports genre:** You play as an individual or a team in a sport. The Wii Sports series is the second-best-selling video game of all time (behind Tetris). EA Sports and 2K dominate the sports games with the Madden Football, FIFA, and NHL series.

Role-Playing Games

Role-playing games (RPGs) are rooted in the Dungeons & Dragons tradition. Players are cast in the role of one or more adventurers who have a specialized skill set. You progress through a story or can play in real time. You may play as a team or be a part of a guild. You can customize your character. (The most well-known RPGs are World of Warcraft and Final Fantasy 14.) RPGs can immerse the player in a new world and be identity forming and all consuming. MMORPGs (massively multiplayer online role-playing games) allow hundreds of players to interact and play together in real time. RPGs and MMORPGs are worth singling out as we try to better understand the gaming world. Stephanie, a high school student, explained to me her experience with World of Warcraft, an MMORPG that has over 40% of the market share of role-playing games:

"World of Warcraft is a huge part of my life, and I got very involved in my guild. I had pretty armor that reflected my skill. I could collect and ride crazy animals. I liked my guild, which is the group of people that I played with regularly. We each had roles and took orders from the guild leader. The guild let in younger players like me, but we had to be polite, and there was a sort of etiquette that you needed to learn. We got to know each over time, and I could get lost for hours in different battles."

RPGs are identity and community forming for both teenagers and adults. Teenagers join "teams" and make strong connections to others online. Guilds have been known to have real-life meetings. Guilds have fostered real-life friendships and relationships. More on these games in Part II of this book. Now that you have the video game road map, let me try to decorate the landscape with some debates and details.

Be a Gamer, Save the World

My 9-year-old son is addicted to video games. He plays on my phone, the iPad, the Wii, and his DS. I can't keep up with his game du jour. Recently he started playing Minecraft. He builds complicated structures with rudimentary blocks. He occasionally kills a zombie and someone makes a crude comment. But in the creative mode, he spends hours building intricate buildings. He threw away his Legos and blocks years ago, but he is transformed into an architect and city planner in Minecraft. It is all consuming and very time-consuming. I can't decide whether to cry or cheer him on.[14]

This mom reflects the ambivalence that comes with video games. Minecraft is my poster child of the new world of gaming. It combines the mindless zombie/monster genre with true creativity. There are limited instructions, and kids have to figure out how to find tools and build structures on their own. The graphics are basic, and the screen looks like Legos, but kids can build whole worlds. There are Minecraft clubs and classes popping up in Europe and the United States.

But all video games are not created equal. When it comes to digital technology, parents of young kids worry the most about video games. They fear that their kids will become "addicted" or exposed to excessive violence.[15] Video games are here to stay, and we are finding the positive effects of video games everywhere. Some game researchers are reporting that games fill genuine human needs that the real world fails to satisfy. In addition, gamers are beginning to use games to solve the real problems of our world.

In 2010 more than 57,000 gamers were listed as coauthors for a research paper in the prestigious journal *Nature*. The gamers, who had no previous experience in biochemistry, were enlisted to work in a 3D game environment called Foldit. In this program, they folded virtual proteins in new ways that could help cure cancer or prevent Alzheimer's. The game was developed by scientists at the University of Washington who believed that gamers could outperform supercomputers in this creative task. The researchers were right. The gamers beat the supercomputers at more than half of the game's challenges.[16]

Jane McGonigal, a game developer and writer, created a game entitled EVOKE for the World Bank Institute. Nineteen thousand players undertook real-world missions to improve food supply, increase access to clean energy, and end poverty in 130 countries. After 10 weeks, they founded more than 50 real new companies still operating today. Her favorite company is called Libraries Across Africa, which has recently been renamed Librii. It is a new franchise system that encourages real book and digital libraries throughout Africa. In her *New York Times* bestseller *Reality Is Broken*, she writes that young people who understand the power of video games will be creating and shaping the future.

SOCIAL MEDIA SERVICE PLATFORM

Social media sites are part of the social media service platform. Social media is a huge part of the digital landscape. I have labeled the diagram on page 72 a "social networking map" to give you a sense of how social interactions connect different platforms and bring our digital landscape together. Social media is defined as a form of electronic communication through which users create online communities to share information, ideas, personal messages, photos, videos, and other content. Social media sites require Web-based and interactive technology platforms to make them work. There are six different types of social media: collaborative projects, blogs, content communities, social network sites, virtual game worlds, and virtual communities.

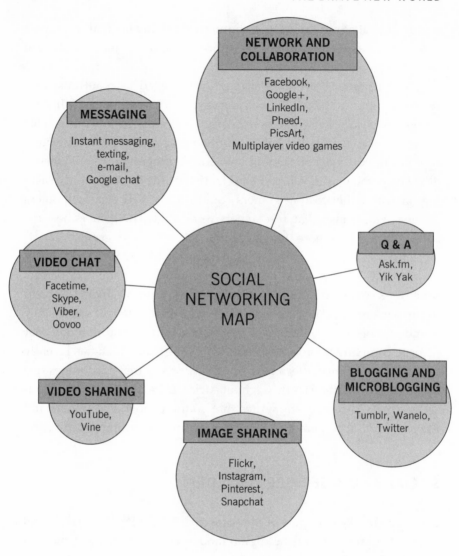

Social media use explodes between the ages of 11 and 14 years. The four most popular social media sites for teens as of 2014 are Facebook, Twitter, Instagram, and Snapchat. Facebook is by far the most popular social networking site worldwide. Facebook exceeded 1.1 billion users in May 2013. If Facebook were a country, it would be close to tying India as the biggest nation in the world with 1.2 billion residents. However, Facebook is quickly falling out of favor with teenagers and young adults. It still occupies a huge piece of digital real estate but is not the future of social media for children and adolescents. In 2013, Twitter briefly took over as the most important social media site, but Instagram took the lead in 2014.[17] However, Snapchat is the fastest rising social media site, especially for younger teens. There are now approximately 500 million users on Twitter, depending on how you define *users*. Twitter is a social networking and microblogging site that enables users to send and receive "tweets," which are text messages limited to 140 characters. Instagram is primarily a photo-sharing site and Snapchat allows users to send images that "disappear" in 10 seconds or less.

Social media use seems to follow a clear developmental path. It starts with simple texts, e-mails, trades, and games. It evolves into the photo- and video-sharing sites such as Instagram and Snapchat. When kids are able to read and exercise even a rudimentary level of typing, they are ready for their first online social interactions. By age 7, kids are old enough to e-mail and play games. From there, they can participate in websites and games online that allow them to play and communicate with others in cyberspace.

My young sons first got excited about social interactions online through fantasy football. The teams compete against other teams in their group. They followed their scores and sent trades through their father's e-mails. Club Penguin, Everloop, and Webkinz are examples of virtual communities designed for 7- to 10-year-olds. On Disney's Club Penguin, kids build igloos and search for accessories. If they amass enough virtual coins, then they can buy "puffles." They can meet their online friends in their virtual communities. Similarly, kids can build and share the creations on Minecraft, and young girls can join Sweety High. Sweety High is recommended for 10-year-old girls. It is a school-themed social network site where girls can interact with friends, earn rewards, and watch the Web series *Sweety*, about three BFFs (best friends forever).

The biggest entrée into grown-up social media is through Instagram and other picture- and video-sharing programs. Instagram has become the "Facebook" of middle school. Instagram is an online photo-sharing, video-sharing, and social networking site. Parents should know that Instagram photos can be shared on Facebook, Twitter, Tumblr, and Flickr.

Since Facebook is no longer "cool" for kids, it is important to understand what is taking its place. In 2012, almost half of kids surveyed considered Facebook the most important social media site. By 2013, that number had dropped to a quarter of all surveyed. As Facebook declines, Twitter, Instagram, and Snapchat are becoming increasingly important.

Beyond Facebook

Other important social media sites that you should know are listed below.[18]

- **Ask.fm:** This social media site allows users to ask and answer questions both anonymously and not. It has become a notorious breeding ground for intimidation and cyberbullying.
- **Google+:** Google's social network was intended to improve on Facebook's friend concept by using "circles" to help users control whom they share with. It's more popular with adults than kids.
- **Instagram:** The most popular social media site among younger teens. The site allows users to snap, edit, and share photos. Instagram is now owned by Facebook.
- **Kik Messenger:** This alternative to texting is available via app. Users often consider it faster and more fun than SMS texting.
- **OoVoo:** With this free video, voice, and messaging app, users can have group chats with up to 12 people.
- **Pheed:** Pheed is an increasingly popular social media site for teenagers. Users personalize their "channel" and can share text, photos, video, and audio notes. Users can share content on Facebook and Twitter. Most people use Pheed like a social media site, but your channel can be monetized. In theory, you can charge users to view your content.
- **Snapchat:** With this messaging app, users can send pictures and videos, putting a time limit of 1 to 10 seconds on how long they last before they "disappear." Snapchat is one of the fastest-growing social media sites. Forty-six percent of teens and young adults have used Snapchat.
- **Tumblr:** This is a cross between a blog and Twitter in which users make their own "tumblelog" of text, photos, and videos that can be shared and followed.

- **Twitter**: On this social network and microblogging site, users can post messages of up to 140 characters (tweets).
- **Vine:** Twitter owns this social media app, which allows users to post, watch, and share looping 6-second videos.
- **Wanelo:** "Want, Need, Love" combines shopping, fashion blogging, and social networking. You can present your own style through the "My Feed" function.

GENERAL TRENDS IN THE DIGITAL LANDSCAPE

The landscape is always changing, but I want to point out some noticeable trends to keep an eye on over the next few years.

- Everything is becoming more mobile.
- Devices are being marketed directly to and designed specifically for kids (i.e., Kurio, Nabi).
- Kids are moving away from Facebook to sites that their parents are not already on.
- Social media starts with picture-sharing sites.
- Kids are very interested in Q&A sites like Ask.fm and "disappearing" sites like Snapchat.
- Hacking and coding are cool.
- Social media has become a platform for social change. There are many ways to give back (e.g., Upworthy, DoSomething).
- My favorite new prosocial and time management app is the Unicef Tap Project. For every 10 minutes you don't touch your phone, UNICEF Tap Project donors can fund one day of clean water for a child in need. Go to *tap.unicefusa.org*.

Having a bird's-eye view of the terrain is a good start toward knowing how you want your family to use digital media. But it doesn't give you everything you need to make informed decisions. The next chapter gives you an understanding of the hot topics debated at school and sporting events, at parties, in the news, and wherever digital immigrants gather.

4

From the iPotty to Facebook Fame

The Good, the Bad, and the Ugly of the Digital Debates

Why did the Flappy Bird developer pull the game?

Are teenagers over Facebook?

Should the NSA have access to our search histories?

Does Beyoncé or Justin Bieber have more followers on Instagram?

Whether you are chaperoning a 12-year-old slumber party, standing on the sidelines at a soccer game, or bidding at a fundraising auction, digital technology will be there. Our national and international dialogue is full of discussions and debates about digital media. It is hard to keep up. As I write this chapter in February 2014, the *New York Times* is covering the bankruptcy of (ironically) a Japanese bitcoin (virtual currency) site, a federal court ordering YouTube to take down a controversial anti-Islam video, and a new educational game company that describes its games as "so much fun that kids don't see the spinach." As a parent, it's imperative that you know the definitions and debates that decorate the digital landscape of the 21st century. You already know a lot of the questions, but the answers will keep changing because the devices, media, and apps are constantly changing. Of course, the questions—those listed above being good examples—will evolve too, as games come and go, pop stars fade, and sociopolitical issues enter and depart the collective dialogue. In this chapter I describe the points being debated as this book is being written, giving you an overview of the issues you'll find examined throughout this book.

WHEN, WHAT, AND HOW?

Cocktail conversation reflects our national or international consciousness on a subject. Daily, I hear adults and kids debating the when, what, and how of technology.

- When is it appropriate for a child to receive or use certain devices?
- What devices should be given?
- How should the devices be managed, introduced, and used?

The *When* Debate

I will be expanding on the *when* debate throughout the rest of this book. The bottom line is that you need to take a developmental approach. Is your child ready for this type of device? Will he be able to use it as a tool? And does he need it at this point? The most hotly debated *when* question is **"When do I give my child a phone?"** If you answered yes to the three questions just posed, then it may be time to buy a phone. Like walking and talking milestones, digital milestones operate in a range of ages. Children generally walk between the ages of 9 and 18 months. Children who walk at 18 months are just as likely to be Olympic runners as those who walk at 9 months. The same is true for digital milestones. Children can develop the tech savvy and skill they need to excel in the digital era whether they are the first or last in their class to get a phone. An 8-year-old with divorced parents who travel a lot might really need a phone. The phone might allow him to move between homes and to speak to noncustodial parents. It might add a layer of safety if this child has multiple pickups and dropoffs with different parents and caregivers. On the other hand, a 12-year-old boy whose mom picks him up and drives him to his activities might not need a phone yet. The 12-year-old boy may be able to e-mail, do homework, and play Minecraft on the home computer. Will both boys eventually get phones? Yes. The *when* debate needs to take a thoughtful, personal developmental approach that reflects the realities and culture of your particular family.

The *What* or *Which* Debate

My 10-year-old niece, Hope, got a smartphone for her 11th birthday. She bought an Android device because the salesman made a great pitch about its versatility. She soon found that her 6th-grade friends all had iPhones and had set up a group chat that was not fully supported by Android. She saw only some of the texts and had difficulty participating in the group conversation. She missed out on a slumber party and didn't know that the group was auditioning for a new play. Is this a life tragedy? Of course not. But it wasn't easy for Hope. She had picked out the wrong expensive device, and her parents were unwilling to immediately buy her another expensive device. Figuring out the "right" age and then deciphering which device or apps to purchase is complicated.

Parents are constantly asking which social media site is most appropriate for their children. Instagram has become the default social media site for middle schoolers, but legally you are required to be 13 years of age to join. The "disappearing" and "anonymous" social media sites complicate the debate further. Ask.fm asks for anonymous comments, and on Snapchat you send images that disappear in 10 seconds (unless they don't). As of early 2014, Yik Yak was the newest culprit. Yik Yak encourages anonymous posts using an alias. The site claims that "what happens on Yik Yak stays on Yik Yak." However, Yik Yak knows your location, and the company has helped the police identify users.[1] I am constantly asking teenagers to ask themselves why they need their images to "disappear" in less than 10 seconds.

> Be a critical consumer: you and your children need to ask yourselves thoughtful questions before spending money on toxic social media sites and poorly designed games and apps.

The list of apps, social media sites, and games that can be downloaded is endless. Parents often get more overwhelmed than their kids. It is critical that parents look at ratings and go to *www.commonsensemedia.org* and read their reviews. Families need to create a continuous dialogue on devices, sites, apps, and games. Children, tweens, and teens need to be enlisted to teach their parents about the pros

Rich Kids' Toys: Privilege or Right?

There are multiple debates about privilege and technology. In the first decade of the 21st century, there was much concern that technology would lead to a further rift between the rich and the poor. Actually, technology has begun to close the gap, not widen it. Technology has become cheaper and more widely available worldwide. Cell phones can be found in some small African towns with almost the same frequency as on Madison Avenue. American researchers have found that lower-income families actually own more devices than richer families. The explanation is that lower-income families may refurbish and recycle multiple devices while richer families simply trade in for upgrades.

The public schools' commitment to technology in the classroom is critical to allow lower-income students to develop the same technology skills as their richer classmates. In the fall of 2013, former New York City mayor Michael Bloomberg launched WiredNYC to bring high-quality free Internet access to public spaces and buildings. WiredNYC is part of a larger national initiative to keep American cities competitive in the business world, but it also serves to democratize Wi-Fi access.

Increased access to technology by lower-income families does not change the fact that smartphones, tablets, gaming consoles, and computers are very expensive, and this factor certainly comes into play in *what* and *when* questions. About once a month, I have a distressed tween or teen in my office lamenting over how she will tell her parents that she lost her smartphone or dropped it in the toilet. Most middle- and upper-class kids expect that they will get a smartphone and a computer. My 9-year-old son asked me if he could get an iPhone for his 10th birthday. I told him that he had to wait until he was 11 years old. He did some calculations in his head and said that he and his brother and sister would have exactly the same phone. I was confused about his logic since his sister is only 5. He explained that he is 9 and that he has 7- and 5-year-old siblings. Since you get an upgrade *every 2 years*, eventually they would all be on the same schedule. It dawned on me that he is years away from his first smartphone but already expects a biennial upgrade.

We need to teach our children that being a digital citizen means respecting expensive devices. From early childhood, children must understand that it is a privilege, and not a right, to own and use digital technology.

and cons of each purchase. Kids and their parents need to be critical consumers and ask themselves the right questions before they spend money and time on toxic social media sites or poorly designed games.

The *How* Debate

I am sure that you have already had this debate with your children, friends, or family. How should technology be introduced, used, and monitored? It should be introduced in a gradual way where more features or apps are introduced over time. The devices and sites should be seen as **tools** and not mere entertainment. Lastly, the devices, the electronic communication, the games, and the Internet use must be monitored. The Kaiser Foundation found that 16% of teenagers had time limits for TV and 26% had rules about the content of the shows.[2] These numbers are way too low. There should always be guidelines. Technology is an extension of your family culture. Your children should understand the basic guidelines with which you approach it so they can internalize them over time. Guidelines should become more flexible over time. Independence should be fostered, but kids should always know that there are guidelines, expectations, and monitoring.

IDENTITY

Being Popular on Facebook Is Like Being Rich in Monopoly[3]

The debate about social media's effects on the social lives of our children and teens rages on . . . and on. It's true: Facebook friends and Instagram followers are not "friends" in the old-school sense. This doesn't mean, however, that true friendship is dead. It does mean that society expects tweens to remain in constant contact with every acquaintance. When I was growing up, there was a joke that there were only six degrees of separation between Kevin Bacon and any A-list celebrity. Most savvy tweens and teens can beat out Kevin for connecting to acquaintances of acquaintances. And most savvy teens know the difference

It is OK to be "popular" on Facebook as long as you choose your real friends over Facebook fame.

between "Facebook friends" (social media followers) and real friends. Still, it is easy to get consumed by social media.

Debates about whether we should get rid of social media are out of date and pointless. Social media is here to stay, so the issue now is how to help kids have good social lives and healthy friendships with social media networks in the mix. For parents, it's important to know what effect social media responses are having on a teen—not so they can decide whether to ban it from their home but so they can provide the perspective about it that some teens may lack.

It is critical that tweens and teens not judge themselves based on the number of followers they have or how many people "liked," "loved," "or "pinned" their posts. Parents also need to be alert for whether Facebook and Instagram are making their teen feel left out or unpopular. But parents can help their teens understand that the ability to amass followers on social media is more about time spent and technical skill than about worth or friendship. It's important to weigh the risks and benefits for each individual child. Instead of banning social media use until your daughter reaches age 16, you might consider whether she can use it as a tool to make plans with her "real" friends. If your 15-year-old son is painfully shy but has a lively virtual social life, think about whether these networks are actually giving him self-confidence. Or is it the opposite? Kids with poor social skills and low self-esteem are less likely to reap the benefits of social media and cyberspace and may be more vulnerable to being hurt, so it's these children who may need extra monitoring and guidance. (I talk more about these children in Chapter 11.)

On the positive side of the debate, the Internet and social media allow teens to explore different identities and forms of self-expression. Again, the question is not whether but how. Can your teenagers learn to express their real selves in cyberspace, and in a way that they can live with years down the digital highway? Can they recognize that most people present highly polished best selves online, as if they're putting together a résumé that will get them the job of their dreams, and resist judging themselves negatively in comparison or being crushed with envy? Self-presentation on social media has become a full-blown area of research. Current findings suggest that those with good social skills and a positive self-image can use social media to strengthen their relationships and their self-esteem. The flip side is that teens and young adults with poor self-esteem and weak social skills may not be able to utilize social media in a helpful way. As a parent, the goal is to help your child connect with real friends on social media and to help your youngsters learn to be critical consumers of social media. I am constantly reminding teens and adults that you can't believe everything you see on Instagram or Tumblr. Social media sites are wonderful places to scrapbook memories and express opinions and likes. They provide a rich opportunity to connect with friends, but they mustn't be taken too literally.

Oversharing has become a hot topic and is the biggest problem that I see for these teenagers. The anonymity and speed of cybercommunication make it too easy to give out too much information. As digital immigrants who are finding their way in this new land, you might instinctively know that your Facebook "friends" who post the details of their PMS symptoms or colonoscopy are oversharing. Your teen, so fluent in digital-speak, may not. Understanding when and where to reveal personal or sensitive information is a learned skill.

> Identifying the right time and place to reveal personal or sensitive information online is a skill that teens have to learn.

Kids (and adults) with poor self-esteem will go to social media to seek reassurance. They will post that they are feeling bad and hope to get encouragement from "friends" and "followers." Some kids will go to Ask.fm, which is a social media site set up in a question-and-answer format. An extraordinarily bright young woman who overshares told me that it took her 50 questions on Ask.fm before she got "hate." She was very excited to get so much positive feedback before the negative. Sites like Ask.fm and Yik Yak encourage oversharing, and kids are routinely harassed and bullied. Yik Yak actually taps into your GPS. Kids can post comments about anyone within a 10-mile radius. Social media should be used as a place to get advice and support from friends, not hate and harassment. Parents must help their children cultivate the skill to share and seek reassurance in a restrained and appropriate way.

Selfies or Self-Absorbed?

The Oxford English Dictionary's naming *selfie* the official word of 2013 has sparked a debate about whether this generation is too self-absorbed. Selfies taken in moderation can be a whimsical and creative form of self-expression. They can be quickly posted or texted to convey a feeling or document a moment. Selfies have become digital memes more than expansive photo albums. A meme is an image, word, or phrase transmitted from person to person within a subculture to convey a joke, thought, or idea. Most kids selfie and post often, but kids who fear selfies or can't choose a selfie may be confronting more serious body image and identity issues. Life is more than a series of perfect selfies. All kids should be encouraged to use selfies in moderation and to remember to enjoy and experience the current moment rather than merely recording it.

Selfies are a perfect example of how communication has changed thanks to digital technology. In his Pulitzer-nominated book *The Shallows*, Nicholas Carr writes about how the Internet has changed our brains as "written" communication has evolved into a shorter, more visual modality. Parents worry about whether the meteoric shift from the written tradition to the tweet/text tradition is threatening literacy. There is no question that digital technology, from emoticons to selfies, is changing the way we read and write. A 15-year-old ninth-grade boy explained to me that he learned grammar and etiquette online. He moderates a role-playing forum where he develops a story and setting, and others on the forum submit character profiles for consideration. He chooses the writers who he feels have the best grammar and social etiquette so the story will flow the way he envisioned it. His online collaborative storytelling contributes to his literacy, grammar, creative, and writing skills.

A British study found that use of textism (the language used in text messages) was linked to improvement in reading and spelling. They found that texting by 8- to 12-year-olds helped to improve phonologic awareness, the ability to understand and manipulate sounds.[4] Children and teens will inevitably rely on autocorrect and spell check, but they must also know the time and place for textism versus more formal grammar. Communication has become more complicated and multifaceted. Kids must learn to clearly communicate their intentions via words, pictures, hashtags, or emoticons. Electronic communication and online writing may end up contributing more to literacy than it takes away.

The iBlankie: Sleeping with Your Phone

As I have already discussed in Chapter 2, parents have worried that technology robs us of our sleep since the 1800s. Ironically, the research reports that teenagers today are sleeping almost as much as the previous generation did, but anecdotal evidence says otherwise. Unplugging and shutting down are the hardest part of managing technology. Parents report the most conflict about bedtime and logging off. Digital technology keeps us awake. The backlights on the devices can inhibit the melatonin release necessary for sleep. Highly stimulating games or violent shows can make the transition to sleep more challenging. Devices need to be shut down 30 minutes prior to sleep. However, it is not enough to shut down devices; the devices should not go to bed with you.

It's not enough for teens to turn off their phone or tablet—these devices should go to bed in another room.

Sleeping with your phone has become a national epidemic. Kids are afraid that they might "miss" something when they are asleep. A teenage girl told me that she must sleep with her phone in case any of her friends needed her in the middle of the night. The beeps and chirps of updates and messages hum throughout the night. Adults and kids report feeling "uncomfortable" trying to sleep without their phones. I suggest to parents that all family phones go into a communal charging station that sleeps in a common room. I find it amusing when parents tell me that their children must sleep with their phone because they use it as an alarm clock. The last time I checked, you could buy an old-fashioned alarm clock for less than $10. Don't kid yourself; this is not about an alarm clock. It is about our attachment to our phones. Phones have become like a blankie for older kids and adults. We claim that we can sleep without them and then come up with lots of excuses to sleep with them.

RELATIONSHIPS

Virtual versus Real Relationships

Her is a 2014 Academy Award–winning movie about a man who falls in love with his computer's operating system. He even tries to have sex with her through a surrogate. The director, Spike Jonze, was making a not-so-subtle statement about the changing nature of our relationships. Every day, I sit in my office and hear teenagers say, "He said . . ." and "She said . . ." and "Can you believe he would do that?" I have learned that these teenagers are *never* actually saying or doing these things in person. Most of the time the teenagers are talking about "real" relationships where they physically "hook up" and see each other in person at school. However, almost all of the meaningful communication goes on via text, Skype, Snapchat, or Facebook messaging. They may use the antiquated term "say," but they mean "text" or "Skype." If you think I'm exaggerating, have a conversation with an adolescent between the ages of 13 and 18 and listen to the way she talks about communication with her friends and love interests.

Are we all doomed to fall in love with our computers? Is the beauty of human love dead? Will our children lack the skills to interact with real people? *Of course not.* However, relationships are changing. Parents need to understand that we are dealing with two types of relationships: real and virtual. Both types of relationships have changed. The good news is that kids under 18 years of age are not generally interested in the online dating sites. Most kids prefer human interaction but find texting to be more convenient. The "rules" around dating have changed to incorporate endless texting and often lead to sexting. There is less anticipation, since couples are in constant contact. It is time-intensive. I would argue that it has taken the exciting and painful part of anticipation out of the equation. On the flip side, texting brings down inhibitions. Teenagers can communicate and support each other about real issues related to their relationship and their lives. Research suggests that teenage boys are more able to talk about their feelings via text and subsequently get much-needed support and feedback. The authors of the famous (or infamous) 1995 book *The Rules* have had to rewrite their book with "new rules" to incorporate digital technology.

Parents must also understand virtual relationships. Teenagers are connecting and developing meaningful friendships and other relationships with people they meet online. Is it all bad? No. Throughout this book, you will see examples of how virtual relationships help teenagers feel more connected. Many of the teens I work with report feeling better understood by their virtual friends—these are the people they go to for feedback on their poetry, to collaborate on a project, or to put together a team for a multiplayer game.

> Cooper, age 17, is very bright but not doing well in school. His parents bring him to see me because they fear he is too socially isolated. He spends most of his time in his room on his computer. He is a cute boy who looks younger than 17 years and makes fleeting eye contact. He perks up when telling me about his latest fantasy game and gets bored when I ask him about the SATs and college. I ask him about his friends. He replies that of course he has friends. I ask him if he ever *sees* his friends, and he says yes. I explain that his parents report that he never leaves his room, so how does he see his friends? He rolls his eyes and looks at me with disdain. He sees them online. He goes on to explain that he connects with his school friends online and not in person. His closest friend, whom he has "known for years," lives in Canada, and Cooper says that by my definition he doesn't "see" him but that he is an "old" friend who collaborates on games and projects with him.

This type of conversation is likely familiar to anyone with older teenagers who are very plugged in. We know that quality of friendships is related directly to adolescents' sense of well-being. Most kids and adults prefer real interaction versus online. However, the current generation of young people recognizes the role of virtual friends in their evolving social networks. Digital natives "get" this type of relationship and are truly perplexed at what their parents are so worried about.

What parents are worried about falls into two categories: whether their teens will be safe and whether virtual relationships will replace real human interaction. **Teenagers must understand the safety concerns of virtual relationships.** I generally discourage any virtual relationships prior to high school, but teenagers must be reminded not to give out personal information and recognize that people lie, impersonate, and misrepresent themselves online at times. I do not think that teenagers should ever meet their virtual friends in person unless their parents are involved.

When I meet a teenager who is too dependent on virtual friends, we immediately examine why the teen can't get her social or emotional needs met in the real world. The debate is not whether teenagers should have virtual relationships but how to balance them and use them to augment real-life human interaction. The goal is not to fall in love with your computer but rather to use technology to improve your real-life friendships and intimate relationships.

The Demise of the Phone Call and the Rise of the Text

Traditional phone calls have gone the way of the eight-track tape, the rotary phone, and the dial-up modem. In 2009, the amount of data in texts, e-mail messages, streaming video, music, and other services on mobile devices surpassed the amount of voice data in cell phone calls. In fact, when people do communicate via voice, many are often talking through the Internet. The current trend is to use VoIP-based communication services. Skype, WhatsApp, and Viber are three Web-based apps that allow voice or video chatting through the Internet, often for free.

Texting has overtaken talking, and with the texting revolution has come a whole new style of writing defined by short abbreviations, emoticons, and memes. The average teen sends a few thousand texts per month, and kids struggle with the expectation that they will respond to all of them immediately. So the debate is over how to help them keep up with their friends without feeling overloaded. Parents must help their tweens be kind texters who stay connected to friends while not "hypertexting," oversharing, or being pan-available. Families need text-free time to allow space for homework and human interaction.

Can You Escape Cyberbullying?

Cyberbullying is the use of electronic communication to bully a person. Usually messages are threatening or intimidating. Cyberbullying can include mean texts, e-mails, or photos. In Chapter 9, I will give you examples of how cyberbullying has led to depression and suicide. Almost half of all kids report having been bullied online. Cyberbullying is insidious because you can't hide, but the bully can. It follows you home and lives with you 24/7. The bully may pretend to be your friend or pretend to be someone else in your life. Schools have always struggled with how to manage bullying, but cyberbullying is even more difficult because it doesn't generally happen at school. When learning about digital citizenship, children must learn to identify mean behavior and learn how to stand up to bullies. Parents must provide an open enough environment that kids can come to them when they feel at all uncomfortable online. Families and schools must instill the idea of standing up to cyberbullies and not being passive bystanders.

> Cyberbullying is insidious because you can't hide, but the bully can.

Is Digital Technology Destroying the Family?

Catherine Steiner-Adair's *The Big Disconnect* and Sherry Turkle's *Alone Together* lament that technology is pushing us farther apart. Throughout history, there have been natural and man-made forces that have pulled the nuclear family apart. The truth is that you have to work very hard to keep a family together emotionally and physically. Three- and 4-year-old children engage in what is called parallel play before they learn to play together. Family members are often "alone together" when they sit side by side "playing" in parallel on their devices. As we discussed in Chapter 1, it is your family culture that will determine whether technology is the grease that causes your family to slip away or the glue that holds them together. I encourage family members to take an interest in each other's digital lives. Learn to play a Wii game even if you are terrible. Let your kids show you funny videos on YouTube. Joint media engagement with younger children teaches them about technology and provides for a meaningful human interaction. With teenagers, texting may keep you involved and up to date. With older teenagers, texting may be a wonderful way to stay connected. It allows for a more immediate sense of being involved in their

> Want to keep digital technology from pulling your family apart? Take an interest in each other's digital lives.

lives. You don't need to wait for a Sunday phone call; you can hear about the little details. However, there should be space and time to unplug and connect to each other. Family meals without technology are a good start toward keeping the family together. Parents must be willing to unplug if they want their children to do the same. Regardless of your digital fluency, parents are the most important digital role models. If Mom and Dad can turn off their phones and find time for their families, their children will follow suit.

ORGANIZATION AND INTELLIGENCE

Technology in the Classroom: From Day Care to Dissertation

You can run, but you can't hide. You can restrict technology, but it is in the classroom by nursery school. In the next three chapters, you will see that technology does enter the classroom before diapers leave it. There is a lot of debate on this topic, but it changes weekly. In Chapter 6, I introduce you to the Digitods, the name given to toddlers living in the iPhone age. These kids are growing up during the touch-screen revolution. By the time they could pick up a Cheerio (approximately 9 months), they could pinch and swipe.

Should infants be given smartphones and tablets? Of course not, but we are not as far off as you might think. The AAP does not recommend technology prior to the age of 3. After age 3, it recommends up to 2 hours per day. The key to this *when* debate is viewing **technology as a tool**. It can be a tool to record a puppet show or a tool to explore outer space from the eyes of an astronaut. Whether in the living room or the classroom, we want to teach our children that they don't need technology to understand a geometry lesson, but they may use it as a tool to broaden their understanding by seeing the shapes in a more three-dimensional modality.

The debate on how and when to use technology specifically in the classroom rages on. Technology in the classroom does not need to detract from real-life play, problem solving, and discourse, but again, it should be there as a tool—not for the mere sake of having it. At this

> If we learn everything that we need to know in kindergarten, then we better get cracking on digital citizenship.

transitional time schools tend to be a bit inconsistent and disorganized in their approach. On the one hand, it makes perfect sense for schools to have their own server and post homework in a systematic way that includes parents and students. How to uniformly and thoughtfully integrate technology into their curricula is a more complex issue. Five years ago, schools boasted of using laptops in high school. In 2014, there is lively debate about how to use tablets in nursery school and kindergarten. The director of my daughter's nursery school explained to me that she was trying to introduce digital citizenship in her classroom for 3-year-olds. Toddlers use technology, so it is never too early to teach them digital kindness. If we learn everything that we need to know in kindergarten, then we better get cracking on digital citizenship.

Is Technology Rotting Your Child's Brain?

Technology has to be "rotting" your child's brain, if you believe everything you read. Technology *is* changing our brains. Technology is also changing the way we research, write, and communicate. Life experiences shape and prune our neuronal pathways. Therefore, the brains of every generation look different from those of their parents. Our children's brains may become more skilled at scanning, skimming, and switching. Researchers have found that video games improve visual–spatial thinking and encourage independent problem solving. Inevitably, kids will communicate and write differently. Children have easy access to information. What they need to learn in school is how to assess the credibility and authenticity of websites and how not to plagiarize other people's work. Millennials and Digitods must learn how to use hyperlinks, digital images, video, and special effects when writing a "paper" or doing a presentation. Technology is changing how we write, research, read, and learn but to think that it is rotting children's brains is going a bit too far and is not helpful to our discussion. In general, technology promotes cognitive development when introduced at appropriate ages and in reasonable doses. The early researchers (by early, I mean 1980 to 2008) were very negative about the impact of technology on our brains. Most of that research was about TV and more passive media. The truth is that TV was not found to rot our brains despite early warnings. The biggest negative about digital technology is that it can lead to sedentary behavior. The AAP and every researcher in the field has come out loud and clear that TVs should not be in the bedroom. Many of the newer gaming consoles encourage "exergaming," which is defined as video games that are also a form of exercise. Examples of exergames include Dance Dance Revolution and Wii's NFL Training Camp. Research prior to 2010 doesn't really take into account the interactivity of the current digital landscape.

In general, I am on the side that believes technology has the power to make us smarter. It definitely is not rotting our brains if it is used thoughtfully. I do want to pay attention to the need for real play and the need for deep thought. The same pundits who are saying that technology is rotting our brains are saying that play is dead. I do think it is important for parents to encourage real-life play, especially for young kids. I think technology should never replace play. Life has changed, and kids are not sent out to play in the neighborhood and return at will. Parents need to be mindful of the need for kids to play real games and not only virtual games. Having said that, I believe technology is a huge blessing for play in children over 10 years of age. Multiplayer games, fashion websites, and Minecraft allow older children a socially acceptable place for dress-up, building, and games years after it is cool to play with Lego or Barbies.

Nicholas Carr in *The Shallows* worries about the "death of deep thought." I have my concerns about this as well. Technology is a great tool for problem solving, research, collaboration, and experimentation. However, the Internet does not easily lend itself to deep thought. Knowledge acquisition only goes so far. Great thinkers and high school students alike need time and peace to sit with difficult ideas. The millennials do value the written word, but they want it concise and pithy. Newspapers, magazines, and books are all getting shorter. Articles and ideas are presented in short tidbits. How do we encourage kids to sit with difficult works of fiction or challenging concepts? Scientific discovery generally comes from slow, tedious observation. I believe that this is a real challenge for parents and children. It takes time to struggle through difficult ideas. Throughout the entire book, I encourage families to unplug, alone and together. I want to encourage real interaction, and I want to value quiet time for thought. Our children's brains do look different from our own. They are digital natives, and their brains may be better suited to find space for deep thought amid the chaos of cyberspace.

Is the Internet Causing ADHD?

As a child and adolescent psychiatrist, I find this particular debate to be bothersome. Let me be very clear: **Digital technology does not cause ADHD.** There has been an increase in diagnosis of ADHD over the last 20 years, and there is a perception that there is an increase in the prevalence of ADHD. Actually, the increased number is attributable to better screening by physicians, teachers, and families. There are also improved treatments that have made ADHD a much more manageable disorder. Perhaps to the digital immigrants (like us), our children look distracted and inattentive on the Internet. This does not mean that the Internet causes ADHD. Moderate levels of distractibility are normal. The fact that ADHD medications help with all distraction does not mean that everyone has ADHD. There is interesting research that I talk about in Chapter 11 that links dopamine dysregulation with Internet addiction. Dopamine is also the primary neurotransmitter implicated in ADHD. It may be that the treatments for ADHD can be helpful in the treatment of problematic Internet use. It may also be true that people with ADHD are at greater risk for problematic Internet use. Addiction and ADHD may share a common pathway, but there is no reason to believe that digital technology causes ADHD.

The Myth of Multitasking

The take-home message from the Internet–ADHD debate is the myth of multitasking. We often say that children and adults who have ADHD are poor "multitaskers." However, neuroscientists tell us that "multitasking" doesn't exist. Your brain has to switch from one task to another. Therefore, it cannot attend to two tasks simultaneously. I don't encourage kids to learn to multitask. I want them to understand that multitasking is a myth. It leads to lower efficiency and greater distraction. Digital technology has led to a myriad of distractions that must now be managed. Juggling homework and technology is the biggest challenge for tweens and teens. We need to burst the bubble on multitasking so that we can teach our kids (and ourselves) how to turn off or avoid electronic or Web-based distractions during homework. I think the phone should always be in another room. I think self-control should be a required tool for all students. I am referring to SelfControl software that blocks ingoing or outgoing access to mail servers or websites for a predetermined amount of time. SelfControl can help your adolescent do his homework on the computer without the constant distraction of his favorite social media site.[5] It allows you to blacklist and whitelist sites. Anti-Social is a social networking blocking software program that comes with a preprogrammed blacklist of time-consuming sites. The Anti-Social site boasts that "you will be amazed how much work you get done when you turn off your friends." Since multitasking is a myth and we are worried about "deep thought," parents need to help their children maximize their efficiency and attention when doing homework.

PRIVACY

From Diapers to Death: Your Digital Footprint

After digital citizenship, you need to be able to define digital footprint. A *digital footprint* is the trace that you leave on the Internet. A passive footprint is the information collected about you by others. The active footprint is the mark that you leave in cyberspace. It starts at birth, so new parents should be wary of posting cute baby pictures that could follow your children into the boardroom. Colleges and universities routinely Google prospective students. We all know that prospective employers will check out an applicant's Facebook page and larger digital footprint. For better or worse, young people need to manage their digital footprint.

Unless you are running for public office or head a public company, your digital footprint is not as important as your child's footprint. I have learned that I am a dinosaur. I am in private practice, and people do Google me. I will hopefully have an elegant website by the time this book is published, but at the moment my website states my name and address. People come to me through referrals from other doctors, psychologists, and teachers. My 24-year-old tech-savvy assistant is appalled by my lack of Internet presence, and I am learning the value of improving my digital footprint. I can probably drum up business on the Internet, but my identity and future are not dependent on my digital footprint. This is not true for my children and patients.

There is an upside to a digital footprint. It is an opportunity to present yourself creatively and elegantly. Our children will have large footprints that will hopefully reflect their development, accomplishments, and growth. The challenge for parents is not to be afraid. Your children will smell your fear. The goal is to help your children cultivate a thoughtful and creative digital footprint. They can explore, be silly, and make mistakes. However, they need their digital identity to mirror their real identity. It doesn't have to be a perfect portfolio, but it should be real.

> Your child's digital footprint doesn't have to be perfect; but it should be real and reflect the child's development, accomplishments, and growth.

Not Your Mother's Diary

Privacy may be the most hotly debated topic in digital technology. There are two parts to the privacy debate. You need to protect your children's privacy in the world, and you need to manage your tween's or teen's desire to have privacy from you. Protecting your child's privacy in the world is easier than respecting your child's personal privacy at home. The Children's Online Privacy Protection Act (COPPA) was designed to protect the privacy online of children under 13 years of age. It details how website operators should seek parental consent and includes some restrictions in marketing to young children. It is the reason that Facebook and Instagram require users to be 13 years of age. COPPA has not been found to effectively protect children, since children and website operators can easily circumvent the guidelines. However, it starts the privacy dialogue. At a young age, children need to be educated about the importance of not sharing passwords or personal information. Children should never input personal information without their parents' permission. Children should never share their passwords with anyone other than their parents. Children should seek out their parents' assistance if strangers seek them out online. From the beginning, parents should have all passwords, even if they don't routinely use them as their children get older. Parents need to be the guardians of their children's online safety and privacy.

As a parent it can be tricky to respect your tween or teen's desire for privacy from you. This is a big debate, but I feel very strongly that privacy in the 21st century does not look like privacy in the 20th century. Parents over the age of 30 must be careful not to extrapolate their childhood definition of privacy into the 21st century. The definition has changed. Parents come into my office indignantly stating that they would never read their children's "private" communications. They pride themselves on trusting their children. They had a diary when they were growing up, and they couldn't imagine their parents reading it. The NSA, Google, and Facebook all have access to your child's "private" correspondence. I have a hard time understanding why the NSA should know more about my children than I do.

It is critical that your children understand that **privacy does not exist in cyberspace**. If your tween or teen wants to keep a diary, she can write in an offline Microsoft Word document or in a paper diary with a key (they still sell them). However, once teens post on Twitter or Instagram, their parents need to know about it. Your kids should know that you are monitoring their activity. You should "friend" and "follow" your tweens or teens, but there is no need to officially "comment" or "like" unless you have permission. Your job is to monitor their digital footprint and help them get out of sticky or uncomfortable situations.

"Sexy Ladies": Sex and Sexting in Childhood

Should I be concerned that my 5-year-old daughter is running around the house screaming "sexy ladies," which she learned from the South Korean megahit "Gangnam Style"? It seems that sex and "sexy" are introduced earlier with each generation. Kids use the Internet to find health information. They use it to learn about sex, and they often end up on inappropriate websites. I will talk more about the three-click Google phenomenon in Chapter 9. Basically, the first search is innocent and educational. With each subsequent click, the risk of ending up on violent, racist, sexist, and pornographic sites increases. The truth is that kids don't have to look very hard in popular culture to find sexually explicit content. You can't restrict your children from searching the Internet any more than your dad could successfully hide those *Playboy* magazines under his bed. I encourage parents not to be naive but to talk to younger kids about sex offline before they learn about it online. Kids need to understand that the Internet will provide confusing, contradictory, and sometimes scary information if they haven't acquired basic knowledge from their parents or school. The birds and the bees is a topic for ongoing dialogue that goes way beyond the mechanics of sex (they probably already know that part). In 2015, the "birds and the bees" talk includes body image, consent, Photoshop, violence, and sexting.

Sexting means sending sexually suggestive messages via text or photos. Twenty percent of teenagers have reported sending a sext, and 30% have reported receiving one. I suspect that those numbers are low since most teenagers define a sext as sending a nude or partially nude photo and consider sexually "suggestive" photos and texts to be a normal part of flirting and dating. As a parent, you already know the multitude of risks involved with sexting. Pictures stick around and become a part of your teenager's digital footprint. Snapchat is one of the most common ways to sext. It is a social media site that allows you to send pictures that "disappear" in 10 seconds or less. Teenagers truly believe that they "disappear." However, the receiver can take a screenshot of the Snapchat image. That screenshot can be stored forever and forwarded to whomever.

Electronic communication lends itself to sexting because inhibitions are lowered when the person is not physically in front of you. Selfies and late-night texting make it even easier to cross the line from selfie to sext. Privacy has changed, and electronically sending a sexually provocative photo to a boyfriend or girlfriend is never "private." Of course, peer and cultural pressure plays a role. We live in a culture where most female celebrities market and brand their sex appeal. Sexual peer pressure is not new to teenagers. The biggest difference is that the dumb mistakes that you made in the 1970s and '80s are long forgotten and irretrievable. I encourage teenagers to conduct as much of their relationship as possible in person. I would prefer that they were sexy and intimate in person and not in cyberspace.

Just Take Away the Phone

There is an international dialogue on how to set rules and consequences for using technology. Parents routinely report that the only leverage they have with their teenagers is technology. I often wonder how our parents got us to do anything at all. There was no phone or social media to take away. The debates are really around how much to monitor and how much to "trust" your children. First of all, setting up guidelines at a young age is a critical piece of cultivating digital citizenship and instilling your family value system. A slow transfer of power is recommended, with increased choice and independence with time. Your middle school children must be involved with setting up and understanding rules. Parental controls and filters are fine, but eventually your children will need the independence and judgment to manage technology on their own. I believe that parents should be reading and monitoring texts and e-mails in middle school and social media in high school. There is certainly room for debate about how much to restrict and what to monitor. Harsh restrictions will not prepare your child to use digital technology and may force him or her underground. However, too much "trust" is a mistake because the question is not about trust. It takes guidance and experience to present, post, manage, and navigate technology. We don't expect teenagers to learn to drive on their own. Why should they learn to drive digital technology on their own? Teenagers need a learner's permit before getting a driver's license. I recommend that children get a digital permit until they are ready to drive alone.

> Children don't learn to use digital technology responsibly on their own any more than they learn to drive by themselves.

II GROWING UP DIGITAL

5 Downloading in Diapers

Managing Your Child's Digital World before Preschool

Ages 0–2

My daughter Olivia, who just turned 3, has an imaginary friend whose name is Charlie Ravioli. Olivia is growing up in Manhattan, and so Charlie Ravioli has a lot of local traits: he lives in an apartment "on Madison and Lexington," he dines on grilled chicken, fruit, and water, and, having reached the age of 7½, he feels, or is thought, "old." But the most peculiarly local thing about Olivia's imaginary playmate is this: he is always too busy to play with her. She holds her toy cell phone up to her ear, and we hear her talk into it: "Ravioli? It's Olivia . . . It's Olivia. Come and play? O.K. Call me. Bye." Then she snaps it shut, and shakes her head. "I always get his machine," she says. Or she will say, "I spoke to Ravioli today." "Did you have fun?" my wife and I ask. "No. He was busy working. On a television" (leaving it up in the air if he repairs electronic devices or has his own talk show).

. . . Olivia sighs, sometimes, at her inability to make their schedules mesh, but she accepts it as inevitable, just the way life is. "I bumped into Charlie Ravioli today," she says. "He was working." Then she adds brightly, "But we hopped into a taxi." What happened then? we ask. "We grabbed lunch," she says.[1]

Olivia is 3 and Mr. Ravioli is older, at 7½ years of age, both older than the subjects of this chapter but something of a cautionary tale for those with infants in the family. Olivia is constantly on her imaginary cell phone trying to "mesh schedules" with Mr. Ravioli. Things deteriorate further for Olivia and Mr. Ravioli when Mr. Ravioli hires Laurie to be his assistant. Olivia can no longer get through to Mr. Ravioli, and most of her "interactions" focus on leaving messages for her imaginary friend with his imaginary assistant. No shock—children imitate their parents. Sometimes we truly see ourselves only through our children's eyes and actions. Perhaps Olivia's parents are busy professionals trying to balance a hectic life. Kids begin to model their parents before the age of 3. I imagine that Mr. Ravioli in 2015 would have an iPhone and constantly be texting and posting pictures but rarely available to chat in real time or meet at the playground.

Parents with young babies are the luckiest in terms of digital technology. If you have a child under age 2, you still have an opportunity to manage your own technology habits and lay the groundwork for managing your children's usage. However, there isn't much time to figure out a family plan if you want it in place from the beginning. Children under 2 spend approximately 45 minutes to 1 hour and 15 minutes per day on media.[2] They are predominantly watching TV and videos. The amount of TV has not changed dramatically over the last 10 years, but the way in which they watch TV has changed. Children are more likely to watch delayed TV (DVR, TiVo, On Demand) or Web-based TV. Children of all ages are using mobile devices (smartphones, tablets) with increased frequency.

- 2011: 10% of children under 2 have used a mobile device.
- 2013: 38% of children under 2 have used a mobile device.[3]

The mobile device will be the primary platform for media use for the 2-year-old generation. Why does this matter? The problem with the mobile platform is that it is mobile. It is more difficult to leave it out of the bedroom and the bathroom, and off the dinner table. Two-year-old children are thrilled to go to the playground without their tablets. It is the parents who struggle to keep the devices in their pockets. Mr. Ravioli's goal should be to

> The problem with the youngest kids starting to use mobile devices is that they're *mobile.*

have screen-free time and increased availability for real-life chats and playground playdates. This chapter will help you figure out the right balance.

THE GOOD-ENOUGH MOTHER

Ambivalence seems to be the name of the game in parenting with technology. Janie, the mom of 2- and 6-year-old boys, told me, "My 6-year-old plays Mario Party 8 on his DS while watching Phineas and Ferb on his iPad mini. I worry that he will get ADHD. But he is good at technology and math. Maybe he could be the next Steve Jobs?"

Janie and many other mothers like her worry about whether to restrict in favor of real-life interaction or expose in hopes that their child will become smarter and more prepared. If you approach technology with moderation, you are likely to do little harm either way.

But even more important is to keep in mind the concept of the "good-enough mother," developed by British pediatrician and psychoanalyst Donald Winnicott in 1953. Winnicott believed that mothers needed to provide a holding environment where a baby felt safe and that this environment would eventually expand to extended family and the rest of the world. His theory revolutionized Freudian psychology of the day, focusing on the idea that, to develop an independent sense of self, babies need an ordinary mother who is capable of responding to a typical baby's needs.

The good-enough mother is still a worthy standard. Babies don't need "supermoms"; they need "good-enough" mothers. While our culture loves to blame the mom for whatever befalls her children, the truth is that most parents provide the basics that children need. After that, outcomes are up to genetics and environmental factors that are out of our control. It is critical to arm yourself with the good-enough-mother shield so you can tolerate the disconnect between media recommendations and media reality.

> Don't agonize over what media exposure is just right for your child—remember that being a good-enough mother will serve you and your child well here as it does everywhere else.

GROWTH AND ATTACHMENT: THE DEVELOPMENTAL GOALS OF THE FIRST 2 YEARS

The Hippocratic oath simply asks doctors to "do no harm." The same applies to parents. You will be unable to control your children's destiny (regardless of how hard you try), but you can "do no harm." In the case of the first 2 years of life, this means not allowing digital technology to interfere with the formation of a secure attachment between the baby and at least one primary caregiver. Creating this attachment for your child, along with fulfilling basic human needs, is the primary goal from birth to age 2. Nature takes care of everything else in a normally developing baby.

John Bowlby developed attachment theory in the mid-20th century. The basic premise is that a baby must develop a relationship to at least one caregiver to maximize social, emotional, and cognitive development. Mom and Dad's early responses to and interactions with their baby will shape the baby's attitudes and expectations about the world for the rest of the child's life. Attachment styles develop between 7 months and 2 years. A securely attached toddler will use her mother as support when scared or distressed but be comfortable moving away from Mom to play.

So the real question is not whether digital technology makes a baby or toddler smarter but whether it can aid parents in developing a secure attachment during the first 12–24 months of life. Technology doesn't have to hinder healthy attachment. In fact, a father who uses his own technology to be more efficient may free up more time to be physically and emotionally present with his baby. A mother who is traveling for business can stay more connected by reading a story to her baby using the A Story Before Bed app. The app allows her to customize the story and record it in her own voice. Babies need meaningful human interaction with words and lots of nonverbal gesturing. Babies need their parents to pay attention to them and respond to them. Not all the time. Not even most of the time. **Some of the time.** Baby videos can never replace the value of human interaction in young children.

There is room in your life for both your baby and your phone, but maybe not at the same time.

The challenge for parents is therefore to find the place and time for meaningful real interaction. Parents who are texting, posting, and surfing aren't paying attention to their child even if they're sitting on the floor next to the baby. The baby may have to scream louder and break more things to get parental attention. Or worse, the child may retreat and give up trying to connect with the caregiver. Digital technology has often been referred to as an interruption technology. The iPhone or Kindle can interrupt your time with your baby.

What is the official recommendation for screen time for children under the age of 2?

The AAP has come out loud and strong on media for children under the age of 2. The academy strongly **discourages** the use of any media prior to 2 years of age. AAP updated its recommendation in October 2013 to reflect the realities of media use and to acknowledge the many benefits.[4] However, it couldn't identify any benefits for this age group. A pediatrician on the AAP website put it succinctly: "If a little TV is what it takes for you to get dinner on the table, isn't it better for them than, say, starving? Yes, watching TV is better than starving, but it's worse than not watching TV."[5]

I agree that digital technology offers babies little in the way of social and cognitive development. Digital technology is ubiquitous, however, and it is likely that most babies will be exposed. If you are a stay-at-home parent with one child who has limited obligations outside the home and an around-the-clock staff, then by all means avoid screen time completely. If you don't fit into this category, then be mindful of media choices and use them in moderation—good-enough parenting, doing no harm.

Can I use media to babysit or occupy my child?

Yes. But be honest with yourself about it. Human interaction trumps all media for kids under the age of 3, but if you need to use it sometimes to "babysit," call it what it is:

- **Don't look for "educational" media for this age group.** Zero to 2 is the Hippocratic oath stage. Do no harm or as little harm as possible. The research has found there is neither benefit nor harm in limited, appropriate media in children under 2.[6]
- If the video is for babysitting, limit it to one show and then turn it off. Most kids of the 1970s, '80s, and '90s were put in front of the TV at one point to give their parents a break. There is a big difference between 1984 and 2014. In 1984, *Sesame Street* came

---

 Interaction Is for Engagement, Not Education

Parents often worry about how to enhance their child's development through educational and growth-promoting activities. And many baby experts and websites oblige by talking about creative ways to spend time with your baby. However, I think the Native Americans had it right. They strapped the baby to the mom's back and went to work. They sang and talked to the babies all day long.

I remember being at home with my middle child, Andrew, when he was 7 months old. I was trying really hard not to turn on the TV. At that moment, I really wanted to be one of those moms who sat on the floor and played creative games and puzzles with babies who couldn't even crawl and had virtually no fine-motor skills. It was hard to say whether Andrew or I got bored with peek-a-boo first. I lasted another 5 minutes trying unsuccessfully to roll a ball to him. Exasperated, I put him in the Bumbo (a bright blue foam baby seat popular in 2008) and started reciting the names of every boxed food in my kitchen pantry. As I tidied the kitchen I called out, "Kraft Macaroni and Cheese," "Campbell's Cars noodle soup," "Honey Nut Cheerios," and "Uncle Ben's Instant Rice with chicken and carrots." I sang the names out of tune and made silly gestures and faces about the boxed foods, and Andrew laughed and babbled.

There was absolutely no explicitly educational content in my kitchen pantry, but we were both engaged. We made eye contact, and I spoke to him with intonation and with lots of nonverbal gestures. At that moment, I realized that videos were for babysitting babies and that he and I could just hang out with the TV off. When I ran out of canned food, I turned on *Sesame Street* and called my patient back and checked my e-mail. At that moment, I had found balance between engaging my emerging toddler and finishing my work.

on the TV once a day. It lasted 30 minutes and then it was over. TV doesn't have the same discrete time frame that it had in the '80s and '90s. Today parents have to think about how long they want their child to watch a show or video before they choose to turn it off. The biggest risk is that the TV or iPad will go on and not go off.

■ Set a timer. Most 2-year-olds can figure out how to pinch and swipe another show if you are aren't paying attention.

■ Plan what you'll do during that time. Use the time to do your computer work or to socialize with a friend. Watching with your child is better in terms of attachment building than her watching a show alone, because it becomes an interactive activity rather than a solitary one. However, if you have the time to sit and watch *Doc McStuffins* or *Diego*, you have the time to turn off the video and play a real game or read a real book instead.

> If you have time to watch a video with your baby, why not turn it off and play with a real toy or read a book?

Guidelines for Finding Good Baby Videos

✓ Remember the old standbys, which are still great: can't beat *Sesame Street* or *Dora the Explorer*.

✓ Prescreen videos when possible or use sites like Common Sense Media (see Resources) that provide age-appropriate reviews.

✓ Keep in mind that educational videos are not educational prior to the age of 2.

✓ Say yes to music. Music is wonderful. Choose music that you and your child enjoy. Bach is not making your baby any smarter than Bon Jovi or Madonna.

✓ Try to minimize the advertising.

✓ Also be wary of the advertising claims made for some videos and check them out through reputable sources like Common Sense Media.

How Will Your Baby React to Videos?

- Toddlers 1–2 years of age will respond to familiar and friendly characters.
- Starting at around 18 months to 2 years, your baby may acquire knowledge about colors, numbers, and languages.

Are there any educational videos that would be helpful to my baby's development?

I'll say it again: No. Not prior to age 2. Somewhere between 1½ and 2½ years, children may begin to learn colors and numbers from videos. By age 3, they can definitely grow and learn from educational videos. However, be wary of any claim that a video or show will increase your child's vocabulary, teach her colors, or make her smarter.

I admit it. I was duped by the Baby Einstein craze. Baby Einstein is a company that was started in the late 1990s, offering educational toys, books, and videos to children ages 1–6. Music, math, language, and science were explored through their products. Disney bought the company and created an entire show called *Little Einsteins* that was a mainstay of Disney programming for many years. It was brilliant. Imagine the idea of putting your toddlers in front of a video and—poof!—your baby would become smarter or musically or artistically inclined. Many companies followed suit with Brainy Baby and Classical Baby, but no one dominated the market like Baby Einstein. Julie Aigner-Clark, the founder, was mentioned in President George W. Bush's State of the Union address in 2007. In 2009, the company was estimated to be worth $400 million.[7] At my baby shower in 2004, I received more than a dozen different Baby Einstein products.

Unfortunately, it didn't all add up. It is hard to describe the videos if you have not seen one. They have beautiful music and shift from lava lamps to bubbles to puppets to water.

In 2004, I coordinated a weekly infant psychiatry seminar at Cornell. It was composed of a group of world-renowned early childhood specialists. I told them about the Einstein videos and their purported impact on young children. Dr. Ted Shapiro, former chief of child psychiatry at Cornell and a famous child analyst and educator, asked me how I could believe these videos were educational for my newborn son. Could my son touch the water? Could he feel or pop the bubbles? Did the videos roll the multicolored balls or play peek-a-boo? Did the video provide a real mother to sing songs? Of course not. Babies learn from their mother's touch, voice, and eye contact and not from a two-dimensional video.

Eventually the Baby Einstein advertising backfired. In 2006, the Campaign for Commercial-Free Childhood (CCFC) filed a complaint against the $400 million company alleging false advertising. In the end, the CCFC lost its suit, but Baby Einstein and other similar companies in the United States changed their website and their claims. Disney offered a refund to parents who were dissatisfied, and the last Baby Einstein video was released in 2009.

Julie Aigner-Clark's original company tried to provide thoughtful, age-appropriate programming, and it's important to understand that there is nothing wrong with the videos. But they don't increase language or stimulate brain development in very young children. So the moral is to be wary of advertising. Pick videos that have been well vetted. Use sites like Common Sense Media to help you understand the videos before you buy them.

Oh, and one guideline I didn't list above: buy videos that you might be able to stomach watching with your baby. I have always felt that the brilliance of *Sesame Street* was the occasional joke or image meant for the grown-up. I left my son in front of Baby Einstein alone, but I enjoyed watching *Sesame Street* with him.

Should I read to my baby on an e-reader?

We don't have enough research to say whether there is an advantage to reading on an e-reader versus a real book. There is a lot of nostalgia for the paper-bound book. I happen to share the respect and the nostalgia, but I am not sure it is the future of those born in the 21st century.

If you are using an e-reader with a young toddler, then actually read it to your child. Turn off the professional narration even if the voice does belong to Denzel Washington or Meryl Streep. Your baby benefits from the whole process of reading with a real person. The shared experience is powerful. The audio narration is brilliant when an older toddler is developing independence and phonemic awareness (see the following chapter). Not now.

I have heard early-childhood experts extol the value of holding a book and turning the pages and feeling it. It is true that babies learn kinesthetically. Babies should hold, touch, eat, and feel all kinds of things. I am not sure that it has to be a book. I like the toys, whether in book form or not, that allow for touch and feel, that squeak and sing. I personally like using lift-the-flap books with young children, but I see that children are happy to swipe as well. I will say more about learning to read on an e-reader in the next chapters.

How do I protect my baby from her sibling's digital technology?

I have found that parents of one young child have the technology piece down. They have the child outnumbered and have lots of energy. Stacey is an educated mom of a 1-year-old boy, Spencer. Stacey had a media plan for her oldest son. He had his own portable DVD player with lots of thoughtfully chosen videos. He used his mother's iPad to play educational games about colors, numbers, and music. Stacey and her husband handed him the iPhone occasionally at restaurants but also brought along a bag of crayons, Play-Doh, and wiki sticks. It was all going as planned until Connor was born.

Stacey came to my office anxious and in tears. She was letting both of her sons down. She put Spencer in front of the TV more often because Connor needed a lot of attention. She had trouble being consistent with both Spencer and Connor because life was just more chaotic. Spencer was getting older and growing out of some of the educational shows and games. By the age of 3, Connor was watching movies and playing games that she never ever would have let Spencer watch or play at that age. How could she be losing control when her kids were only 3 and 5 years old?

Stacey struggled with the challenges of multiple children. Some of these challenges are not unique to digital technology. It is more difficult to hover and control things with each additional child. Parents are forced to prioritize and rethink earlier parenting goals. I have found that second, third, and fourth children are often more flexible and accommodating because they have no choice.

The take-home message: It will be impossible to control the media environment of your younger children in the way that you did for your older one.

Suggestions for Digital Technology Use with More Than One Child

✓ Occasionally put the older child in front of the TV to allow yourself to spend some screen-free time with your baby or young toddler. It's OK.

✓ Encourage your older children to watch TV and videos in a more cooperative way with the younger ones:

   ✓ Ask the older children to explain storylines.

   ✓ Ask the older kids to sing songs to the younger ones.

   ✓ Emphasize to your older children the increased responsibility and respect involved in making video watching more of a shared activity.

✓ Encourage your older children to watch some of the little kid shows. I believe that *Sesame Street* is more fun for the 5-year-old than the 3-year-old. The 5-year-old is ready to learn to count and recite letters. He is already familiar with and excited to see Elmo or Big Bird. Don't push your older children into more mature programming.

✓ If a program is truly not appropriate for the younger child, then have your older children watch on mobile devices. There is an advantage to having multiple mobile devices.

✓ Not everything needs to be created equal. You can take along an iPad on a trip for an older child if appropriate but take cars, dinosaurs, and crayons for the under-3s.

✓ Depending on the age of your older children, ask your older children to find appropriate apps and play games or read stories with their

If having multiple mobile devices seems questionable, remember that one advantage is being able to allow your older child to watch on a mobile device something that is age appropriate for him without exposing the younger child to it.

siblings. Older siblings may enjoy the added responsibility of explaining a
story or singing a song with their baby siblings.

> **My husband and I are on our devices all the time. Does this have
> any effect on my baby?**

Yes. A lot of attention is paid to digital technology and babies. Everyone
is concerned about whether to let babies and toddlers watch TV or suck
on the iPhone or play with apps. I have found this discussion to be a
bit misguided. To me, we should be talking about parents' media diets
instead of babies' exposure. Research has shown that young and more
media-savvy parents expose their young kids to more media. It makes
sense. Parents set the tone and model the behavior. Mr. Ravioli is very
busy and overscheduled because that is what Olivia sees in her world.

The "motherhood constellation" is a model that I use to help new
parents make the transition to parenthood. Dan Stern, a famous analyst, suggested that our identity shifts when we enter motherhood and
fatherhood. I believe that this shift includes our digital identities. Parents need screen-free time and need to be aware of the tendency to pull
out the phone or check Facebook when they become bored or nervous.
I spend a lot of time in Chapter 1 asking you to track and understand
your own and your family's media behavior. If you haven't had time to
do that yet, take this simple test: Put away your phone and tablet and
spend 30 minutes with your young child. Don't spend the 30 minutes
chatting with a friend or finishing laundry. Simply sit with your baby
or toddler for 30 minutes. Are you able to sit and be fully engaged? Do
you feel the pull of the smartphone or worry about missed texts? If so,
you will need to practice spending time away from your technology;
see the box on page 113.

Parents often talk about whether they love the "baby" stage or not.
A common excuse for a husband who can't sit with an infant is that he
is not a "baby" type. What he is really saying is that he can't "be" with
a baby who can't interact reciprocally. The baby can't initiate or fully
participate in the play. It can be unfulfilling or even boring to sit with
a toddler who can't play reciprocally. Some parents will hide behind
their technology. Sitting on the ground with the phone or tablet might

Developing Your Tech-Resistant Muscles

The best time to practice is when you most crave your phone or Facebook. Here are some opportune times:

- Try to not look at your phone first thing in the morning: no alarm, no weather, no Facebook update.
- You just sent out an invitation on Paperless Post for your 40th birthday. No checking or peeking to see who responded.
- Your March Madness or fantasy football draw has been posted. Don't look at it until tomorrow (or at least later today).
- You are at dinner with three other adults. One adult pulls out her phone to check something. In digital etiquette, you are now allowed to check your phone. The other two grown-ups reflexively check their phones even though they have not received a ring , beep, or vibrate. Can you resist?

make it easier to tolerate a baby who is batting away at the pack and play. The problem is that the parent is physically present but not emotionally present. I encourage parents to practice being away from their technology and being present with their child. The key is quality time, not necessarily the quantity of time.

EXAMPLES OF QUALITY TIME

- 15 minutes of story time with your baby.
- A 10-minute concert where you sing your favorite 1980s hits.
- A 10-minute tour of the kitchen where you explain in detail how to make macaroni and cheese—even better if the baby can touch the pasta and help pour the water.
- 5 minutes of building towers and knocking them down.
- A 5-minute stuffed animal/puppet show where you tell the story of how you met the baby's mother or the details of last night's football games (get the point—the content matters less than the intonation and interaction).
- 10 minutes of bathtime with lots of messy paints and squeaky toys.

All of these activities are done with the technology carefully hidden in another room. It is quality time—not quantity—that makes the difference.

TAKE-HOME POINTS

✓ Verbal, real-life interaction always trumps screen time!!!

✓ The emotional and cognitive goal of the first 2 years is to develop a healthy attachment to a caregiver.

✓ Educational videos do not stimulate cognitive or social development in children 2 and under.

✓ Music and educational videos watched in moderation do not harm children less than 2 years of age.

✓ Reading to your children is wonderful whether it is on a tablet or paper-bound book.

✓ Videos should be used to occupy babies when parents need a break, not as a substitute for real-life interactions.

✓ Limit the amount of digital babysitting time per day.

✓ Younger siblings may be exposed to more media. Make it as appropriate and interactive as possible. Encourage older siblings to use digital technology cooperatively when possible.

✓ Parents should practice observing 20- to 30-minute screen-free periods for themselves.

✓ Parents should be aware of their own technology diet and modeling behavior.

6 Digitods and Technotots

Everything You Need to Know about the Digital World You Learned in Kindergarten

Ages 3–5

Jennifer, a 40-year-old mother of three, walked into my office worried about technology for her 4-year-old daughter, Addison. She explained that media had been a big part of her childhood. She had watched *Sesame Street* and *The Electric Company*. Her dad was a techie and one of the first to get a Magnavox game console. The Magnavox had a full keyboard console in 1982, but the technology wasn't there, and much to her dad's disappointment, the Atari and joystick technology took off instead. She remembered her dad staying up very late trying to program the computer or playing rudimentary adventure games. She grew up with the utmost respect and fascination for technology but had always relegated it to the sidelines of her busy life. In contrast, at the tender age of 4, Addison seemed to be living in a world defined by technology. So much had changed since the birth of her first son, Harrison. Should she be worried about Addison?

Harrison was born in 2004. He is a digital native and had a Leapster and a portable DVD player by his second birthday. He tried to play Bob the Builder and Dora the Explorer on the Internet. The games were slow and required a mouse or arrow keys to navigate. There were lots of written instructions. His parents had to help him a great deal since he hadn't yet acquired the fine-motor skills to play on his own. He loved the games so much, though, that his parents were willing to play them for him, with his direction. Harrison also watched Baby Einstein and *Sesame Street* videos. He learned to read with board books such as *Goodnight Moon* and the *Biscuit Puppy* book series and didn't see his first YouTube video until first grade. At his Manhattan nursery school, Harrison hung his attendance card on the door in basically the same way that Jennifer had in 1974.

It was a brave new world by the time Jennifer's youngest child, Addison, was born 4 years later in 2008. The family no longer traveled with a portable DVD player because Addison's parents downloaded shows onto their iPad. They bought Addison plastic electronic toys like the Leapster, but those were cast aside in favor of the iPhone, which had much more appeal. By the age of 2, Addison could easily navigate a tablet and had an endless supply of amazing apps. She learned to write her letters by tracing them on Writing Wizard. She counted apples and monkeys on her math apps as soon as she was old enough to speak. Baby Einstein was gone (see Chapter 5), but TV was present. The TV platform had evolved. Addison didn't watch the morning lineup on *Nick Jr.* She picked out her show of choice, and it was played on demand or downloaded onto a tablet or computer. Addison had no concept that TV could be watched in real time. On occasion, she tried to swipe the mounted flat-screen TV and had no interest in the remote control. Jennifer and her husband read to Addison alternately on an e-reader and with real books. Addison read her first book on a tablet. At the age of 5, she can problem-solve on a tablet. She can figure out how to download an app. She can teach herself how to play a game by feel and trial and error. On her first day of nursery school, she dragged a picture of herself on the smart board into an animated image of the school. The first time she had the attendance job in her nursery 3-year-old class, she "FaceTimed" the nursery school director and announced the names of the children who were absent.

If you haven't figured it out yet, I am Jennifer (my middle name), and Harrison and Addison are my oldest and youngest children. I thought it was revolutionary when Harrison started to use technology, but everything changed with the popularity that the iPhone and iPad brought to touch-screen and interactive technology. Addison moves fluidly between the digital and real worlds. She views reading a book on the Kindle or playing Yahtzee on an iPad as merely a choice. Sometimes we play Yahtzee with real dice and sometimes on the iPad. She will pick up the iPad to read a book as easily as she picks up a paperbound book. She plays games on the iPhone but quickly turns them off to play a board game. She prefers real board games, puzzles, and imaginative play. But she will happily play one of her brothers' new games or watch another episode of *Fresh Beat Band*. She views technology like a board game on a shelf—one of many choices. The virtual world and the real world have been coalesced into her own world.

Addison is a Digitod—the designation for children born since the inception of the iPhone in 2007. Digitods have no PI (pre-iPhone) memory. They are the pioneers of the touch-screen revolution. The touch-screen revolution has changed the way we all live, but it has been a true revolution for toddlers. Prior to 2007, toddlers needed to use a mouse or a keyboard to navigate games or the Internet. Literacy was a requirement for full navigation. That is no longer true.

If your toddler resembles Addison, or is a somewhat typical 3- to 5-year-old, she is probably still watching a fair amount of educational TV, cannot yet navigate games and apps that

> Digitods are the pioneers of the touch screen revolution.

require sophisticated language and keyboard skills, but is pretty comfortable swiping a tablet screen. Your Digitod may already be fluent in all kinds of digital tech use if the family is immersed in digital media and you have older children. It's a wide-open frontier for kids at this age, with an incredible opportunity for you to start to form a family plan that will serve you in the years to come. More on toddlers' current use of technology is detailed later in this chapter.

LEAPS AND BOUNDS: DEVELOPMENTAL GOALS FOR TODDLERS

The toddler years have been appropriately described as the "magic years."[1] Three-year-olds are awake and engaged and excited about everything. They believe in magic but also have lots of questions. They are sponges that absorb information from everywhere. Watching toddlers transform every minute can make you feel like all the energy and language they've been bottling up in infancy has just exploded. The physical, cognitive, and emotional development of the 3- to 5-year-old is meteoric. And the days of your being able to control all the variables in your child's life are over (even for those Ivy league–educated professional moms).

Cognitive Development

"Why?" is the mantra of the toddler years. Toddlers' curiosity is boundless. They will learn to solve problems by trial and error, repetition, and observation. Their ability to solve problems improves as their attention span, symbolic thinking, and fine-motor skills develop. Their problem solving will be hampered by their inability to distinguish fantasy from reality and their egocentric approach to the world. Toddlers can truly problem-solve on a tablet. They can recognize an icon for a game or a video. They use trial and error to get something started. They can figure out how to stop, start, and restart a video. They can figure out how to change colors on a drawing app. They will still believe that Elmo is speaking directly to them and that he is gone when they turn him off. However, they can use basic language skills, pattern recognition, and fine-motor skills to solve real problems and begin to navigate the digital world.

While there are many components to toddler cognitive development, parents are stuck on language at this stage. It is normal for parents to count the days and the words that their toddlers say. Parents have been waiting years to have a somewhat meaningful and reciprocal conversation with their toddler. Additionally, language is the first step in the cognitive journey, and good language skills bode well for a toddler's future academic abilities.

Toddlers' language is growing every day. They are able to express real ideas and understand the world outside themselves, although their ideas are still bigger than their vocabularies. It is so common for your toddler to come home from nursery school overly excited. She may be full of energy and jumping from one activity to another. She can't explain all the details of her day, but her energy and enthusiasm give you some sense of her excitement. Usually, toddlers are chatterboxes who imitate the world around them. At 3 and 4, they express themselves through their behavior. They tantrum easily and often because they can't quite "use their words" to get their points across. Toddlers must begin to use language and self-regulation for meaningful self-expression.

Physical Development

Physical development and motor skills are a huge part of toddler development. Of course, your toddler will learn to walk—hence the name "toddler." From the ages of 3 to 5 years, your child will learn to throw a ball, squat, and ride a tricycle. Toddlers develop the motor skills to use a spoon and a cup. Your toddler will want independence and get frustrated when she can't accomplish her goals—thus the toddler temper tantrum.

Here are some general physical milestones to look for:

- Ride a tricycle
- Throw a ball
- Go down a slide without help
- Do somersaults
- Walk backward
- Jump on one foot

There is no reason for technology to hamper physical development, although at this age there isn't much it can do to promote development

How to Protect Your Toddler from Negative Effects of Technology

- No TV or digital devices in the bedroom. It can lead to obesity, metabolic abnormalities, and sleep disturbances.
- Don't leave the TV on when no one is watching (i.e., background TV). It detracts from human interaction and leads to inappropriate exposures.
- Turn off devices at least 30 minutes prior to bedtime. Do not allow your toddler to hold a tablet close to his face prior to bedtime. Late-night technology and background blue light can disrupt sleep and lead to physical, behavioral, and emotional problems.
- Limit junk food advertising. If you can't, then discuss the ads with your toddler and offer healthy alternatives.
- Present your toddler with lots of opportunities to run around and be physically active. Rarely do toddlers choose sedentary behavior if given an alternative. Encourage healthy physical activities and games.
- Present your toddler with lots of opportunities for real-life imaginative play. Play promotes social and emotional development.

either. See the box on page 119 for ways to prevent the use of digital technology from having a deleterious effect on your Digitods.

Social and Emotional Development

Your toddler's temperament and personality may begin to flourish. Temperament reflects certain innate aspects of your personality such as introversion or extroversion. It is usually understood in categories such as activity level, adaptability, intensity, and initial style of reaction. Personality is acquired throughout life on top of your temperament. Family experiences and education can play a role, and personality is composed of beliefs and feelings. For example, your toddler's temperament may make her easy to soothe and sleep but slow to warm up around strangers. However, her personality may be to be loud and persistent so she can be heard over her older brothers. Both temperament and personality will play a role in how your child manages technology. If she is "easygoing" and transitions easily, then unplugging may not be a problem. If she is easily overstimulated and hyperfocuses, then technology may quickly become an area of contention.

Lying and the beginning of peer pressure emerge in toddlerhood. Lying is common and expected as toddlers try to determine the difference between reality and wishful thinking. While toddlers are egocentric, they will begin to develop sympathy and pay attention to the world around them. They will get social feedback that will shape their behaviors. My middle child, Andrew, had a playdate with a friend in nursery school. His friend commented about the nighttime pull-ups sitting on his dresser. In typical boy fashion, Andrew was not in a rush to be dry at night. However, the night after this particular playdate, Andrew was immediately potty trained. A couple whom I treat were distraught that their 3-year-old daughter, Bella, went to nursery school with her thumb in her mouth. Despite all their begging and bribes, Bella was determined to suck her thumb at school. One day in September, during imaginary play, a friend and classmate imitated Bella by putting her thumb in her mouth. Bella came home and said nothing. There were neither tears nor drama, but Bella no longer sucked her thumb at school. She sucked it at night and when she was sick or stressed but not at school. Peer pressure is powerful even in nursery school.

Play: All Important and Ever Present

I rarely go a day without hearing a well-meaning friend, colleague, educator, or parent talk longingly of the "good old days" when you gave kids a cardboard box and a bike in nursery school and off they went, only to return on the first day of first grade. No schedules, no classes, no kindergarten entrance tests, and **no electronics**. Who hasn't bemoaned the overscheduled toddler who doesn't have time to play?

Play is a big buzzword in child development these days. And it should be. Play is super-important. But it is hardly dead, and I am a bit tired of the bereavement over the loss of this part of children's lives.

Just watch your toddler closely for a day and you'll see all the many ways your son or daughter engages in play. Don't be fooled by the fact that toddlers primarily use parallel play. They enjoy counting and sorting. They notice similarities and differences. They like imaginative play. It is a wonder to observe the imagination of a toddler. It is disinhibited, nonlinear, and so much fun. And it is evident in your toddler's daily life, in both planned and directed activities and spontaneous play.

Let's face it: Disney would be in a lot of trouble if play were dead. What would happen to Cinderella, Elsa, or Santa Claus? Fantasy helps toddlers understand the world around them. They are drawn to superheroes and princesses, but they will also emulate and desire toys that mimic various facets of the adult world. I remember buying a light-up pretend cell phone for my older son (2007), a pretend BlackBerry for my younger son (2010), and handing Addison my real iPhone to play with (all in 4 short years).

The goal is to cultivate creativity and encourage parallel play that will soon evolve into reciprocal play and the foundation of your toddler's social world. You can do this with digital and other toys, with active and quiet activities, at home and everywhere else—and, believe me, your child's preschool, day care center, and sports coaches are on it.

THE STATS: ARE TODDLERS REALLY USING THAT MUCH TECHNOLOGY?

I see technology use as having several spikes. The first big explosion is at 3 to 4 years of age, followed by another burst at 8 years old, and a final tween peak in middle school at 12 or 13 years. Technology seems to be somewhat safely under parental control until about 8 or 9. However, the quantity and type of usage change yearly.

> In just the 2 years between 2011 and 2013, the number of kids under age 8 who had used an app had more than tripled— from 16% to 50%.

Every year sees an increase in the time spent on digital technology, the quantity of devices, and the number of ways they are used. Two- to 4-year-olds spend approximately 3 hours per day on screen media, but this will increase to an astounding 7¾ hours by the end of elementary school. At this stage, TV is the primary mode of technology. The good news is that there is lots of educational TV. The bad news is that this will dramatically end by second grade. The biggest transition in the toddler years is that children will shift from passive TV and videos to playing all kinds of games and apps before they start kindergarten. By kindergarten, they will be able to take advantage of the apps and games available on smartphones, tablets, and computers. I suggest that toddlers begin to play games on tablets rather than smartphones when possible. The tablets allow for larger screens and easier navigation. I encourage you to have a family tablet or computer that your toddler can use when she is ready for educational games and books. The pitfalls of toddler usage arise when parents put a TV or computer in their child's bedroom and when they leave the TV on all the time. These days **more than a third of kids between 2 and 5 years old have a TV in their bedroom**— and 10% of kids under age 2! Yet bedroom TV and background TV lead to increased sedentary behavior and inappropriate, extended exposure. **This is the moment to turn off the TV and keep it in the living room.** Your toddler may tantrum, but a toddler tantrum is nothing compared to the inevitable rage of the teenager who does not want technology taken out of the bedroom.

The time spent on various digital media by 2- to 5-year-olds is shown in the pie chart and the bar graph on page 123.

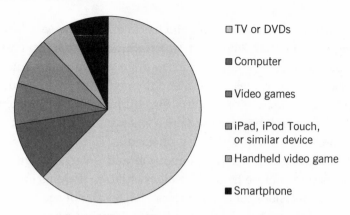

Time spent using screen media, ages 2–5, by medium.
Based on Wartella et al.[2]

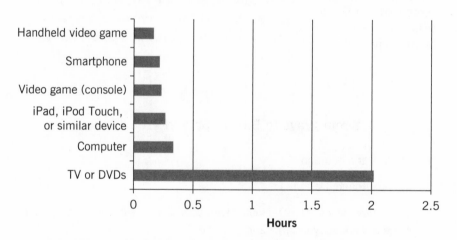

Time spent using screen media, ages 2–5, by number of daily hours.
Based on Wartella et al.[3]

How much time should my toddler spend on technology?

Focus on screen-free time. Don't worry about total time yet! Of course time will vary depending on whether you are a media-light, media-moderate, or media-heavy family (go back to Chapter 1 and figure this out if you haven't done so yet). Birth order also plays a

Parents control most of their kids' exposure to technology before age 8, so the stats on toddlers' use of digital media tell us what parents are allowing.

role in how much exposure your child has to media. The AAP is recommending no more than 2 hours of "entertainment" media for children. The academy's recommendations for toddlers are unclear. As noted in the previous chapter, they recommend no media for children under 2. Their general guideline of 2 hours for children is not a particularly helpful recommendation for toddlers. Generally, toddlers don't spend much more than 2 hours per day on media. The AAP has recently started to distinguish between education and entertainment media. This distinction is more helpful for older children. Parents make most of the media decisions for children less than 8 years of age.

> For toddlers, it's more important to designate screen-free time than to limit exposure to technology.

For toddlers, I focus on **screen-free time** versus limiting overall time. Since adults are controlling most of the exposure, my hope is that parents will have delineated screen-free times when both toddler and parent are off all media (including phones).

Some Ways to Ensure Screen-Free Time

✓ No TV in the bedroom.

✓ No background TV.

✓ Spend intervals of 20–30 minutes with your child without getting on your phone or handing your phone to your toddler.

✓ Model that parents can be engaged and present with their children without digital technology.

✓ Try to limit technology time to one show (approximately 25 minutes) at a time.

✓ If necessary, intersperse TV time with screen-free time for your toddler.

✓ Avoid sitting a toddler in front of the TV for more than 45 minutes at a time.

> **Are tablets and smartphones (like the iPad and iPhone) really appropriate educational tools for my toddler?**

Yes, yes, and more yes. Patti Wollman Summers, author of *Toddlers on Technology*, argues that the iPhone is **the most effective teaching tool since the invention of chalk and the slate board.** Summers, who is an early-childhood educator, reports that kids come into nursery school more prepared for formal learning due to their experience with apps and interactive technology.

The tablet is an ideal learning tool for young children due to its accessibility and ease of use: iPads are interactive, repetitive,

> Tablets teach the way toddlers learn.

and nonjudgmental. They teach the way that toddlers learn and can be operated using the skills toddlers already have. Tablets and smartphones require limited literacy and are easy to navigate. By approximately 1 year of age, children learn to point and use a pincer grasp—the ability to use your thumb and forefinger together. Having a pincer grasp allows you to pick up Cheerios or pinch an iPad screen. Once you can point and pinch you can operate a tablet.

Most apps and games are interactive. They prompt and speak to the toddler. They require toddler participation, which promotes cognitive development and even social development. Like all machines, the tablets are not judgmental. If you miss the task, then you do it over again. Most toddler apps have lots of smiley faces and encourage kids to try again. There is no grandparent or parent asking the 4-year-old to count to 10 in Spanish like Dora or spell the word of the day like Elmo.[4]

> Once your toddler can point and pinch, he or she can operate a tablet.

> **How can digital technology cultivate my child's development?**

Cognitive Development

Both iPads and iPhones are wonderful educational tools for this age group. The Internet can be an incredible place to explore the **"why."** My kids never tire of trying to stump the voice-activated function named "Siri" on my iPhone. More seriously, Addison, now age 5, and I went to *kids.nationalgeographic.com* and named a panda, watched a video about the queen angelfish, and did a static electricity experiment where we used a comb to "wiggle" water. It is so easy to go on a virtual scavenger hunt with your child, exploring animals, music, countries, or whatever catches your interest at the moment. Your toddler can be the navigator, and you can be the driver. You are cultivating curiosity and engaging your toddler in a joint open-ended endeavor.

Take your toddler on a virtual scavenger hunt in which the toddler navigates and you drive.

There are also lots of apps that toddlers can explore on their own. They can point and pinch their way through a game or educational app. They gain experience, mastery, and independence. Educational TV and games can be used to enhance language development at this age. Technology should not replace real-life reading and talking. It is an add-on with no downside if used thoughtfully and in moderation. There are apps that teach kids to trace letters, like Writing Wizard, and to learn letter sounds, like Starfall. My First Tangrams promotes visual–spatial skills with colorful puzzles. Dora and Ni Hao Kai-Lan expose toddlers to foreign languages and cultures.

I will never forget an anxious dad calling me about his very bright 3-year-old daughter, Cassie. He was shocked that Cassie did not know her colors. He had pointed to the sky and asked Cassie the color of the blue sky and she had said, "azoo." He had asked again, and she said, "azoo." I asked him if she watched *Dora the Explorer,* and he quizzically responded that it was one of her favorites. I suggested that maybe "azoo" was actually *azul,* the Spanish word for "blue." He was quite embarrassed, since he was fluent in German and Dutch, but acknowledged that this could be a plausible explanation. Will Dora make you fluent in Spanish? Absolutely not, but there is nothing wrong with exposing young children to foreign languages and new phonemes (the building blocks of language that distinguish native speakers from accented speakers).

Social and Emotional Development

The question is how technology can assist in your toddler's development into a social being. Most social development at this age comes through play, so apps that encourage interaction and imagination can promote social development. For instance, My Play Home is an interactive app that allows a toddler to create a family that lives and plays in a home. Peek-a-Zoo teaches social cues by asking toddlers to identify the feelings and behaviors of the animals. I want to be clear. I believe that technology is an incredible tool for play and creativity at all ages. I think it is a more important tool for creativity and identity development in older children than in younger children because the digital world is a powerful place for older children to try on new roles and characters—a type of creativity that comes more easily to toddlers, who don't need technology to play dress-up or to create music. Toddlers don't "need" apps and technology for play and social development, but properly chosen apps used with parents or caregivers can enhance and enrich your toddler's social and emotional growth.

Technology can be used as one of many tools to cultivate creativity and cooperative play. For example, I love the playful TV musical shows like *Fresh Beat Band* that have lots of singing and silly stories. In *Doc McStuffins*, Dottie McStuffins uses her imagination to doctor her stuffed animals and dolls. It reminds me of the imaginary world of Winnie the Pooh. I also like many of the arts and crafts programs and apps. I try to carry markers and paper when we go out to dinner or travel. When I forget, I open the iPad to Scribble Press or Nick Jr. Draw and Play. Addison also loves to decorate doughnuts, cookies, and jewelry. She mixes colors and adds textures. She can use her art apps to develop an art portfolio that can be shared with her grandparents across the country. Online drawing should never replace real-life crayons for toddlers because physical painting and drawing encourages fine-motor development. But virtual crayons are a fantastic substitution when you leave the markers in the car or when your toddler wants to try something new.

There is also a role for technology in encouraging socialization and cooperation. While toddlers can be mesmerized by a show, they can also work together on a computer program or app. Technology can be a potentially shared experience for a toddler and her older siblings. (More on the subject of siblings is to come later in this chapter and the rest of the book.) Parents often enjoy playing a game or navigating the digital world together.

Should I be worried about violence impacting my toddler's development?

Yes and no. Try to avoid any shows or games with violence. Look at reviews for their description of violence. However, I want to distinguish between TV or video game violence and aggression that is a normal and healthy part of toddler play. When my boys were toddlers, I actually felt like a good mother every time they put on Spider-Man or Jedi costumes. I even encouraged light-saber battles and Nerf gun attacks.

Wait—don't judge yet. I recognize that not everyone agrees, but I wanted to encourage their imaginative play, and I observed with my patients and my children that aggression was a real part of play. I did not allow violent video games or TV shows. I didn't want my kids to get the message that it was OK to hurt someone—*ever*. I preferred that they explore their aggression in their 3D imaginary play and not in their 2D computer play. They got real feedback if they hurt each other and developed a degree of empathy for each other. I believe that real play is a more appropriate place to express the aggression of toddlerhood. It is too early for violent themes to creep into TV shows and games. There is a role for violent video games in safely expressing aggressive urges, and very soon, you will be unable to completely avoid it. But for now I would try to keep the aggression confined to the real play and out of the digital technology.

> Tangible, 3D aggression is a healthy part of toddler play. It allows for a release of energy and hopefully results in the development of empathy. It's preferable for toddlers to have light-saber fights and play cowboys than begin to play solitary, sedentary violent video games.

How do I choose what type of technology my toddler should use?

The developmental progression of media starts with educational TV and progresses to a combination of educational TV and educational games and apps. Later, kids drop most of the educational TV and may or may not continue with educational games. By the end of elementary school, they will likely use technology for school but spend most of their screen time on entertainment and socializing.

Naming Names: What Exactly Is Age Appropriate for Toddler Viewing?

- Embrace the old standbys, such as *Sesame Street.*
- Trust PBS and Nick Jr. programming.
- I generally trust Disney Jr. but would prescreen the shows since these tend to contain more advertising and marketing.
- Cartoon Network and Disney are generally not age appropriate for this age group.
- Kidz Bop changes lyrics of mainstream songs to make them age appropriate.
- Use the Common Sense Media site to get extended reviews of programming.

Toddlers spend most of their screen time watching TV and videos. As described above, thoughtful, age-appropriate programming and games can help your child with social, emotional, and cognitive development. Media can offer educational and prosocial benefits. Studies of *Sesame Street* over the years have found that children who watch the show play more cooperatively, show more tolerance, and choose nonaggressive responses to situations.[5] PBS, Nick Jr., and some Disney Jr. programming aimed at the under-5 group have lots of educational benefits. It is relatively easy to find quality educational programming for the under-5 age group.

How to Pick Good TV Shows and DVDs for Your Toddler

√ Target audience should be children age 5 and under.

√ Show duration should not exceed 30 minutes.

√ Look for 30-minute shows that are broken down into shorter segments.

√ Avoid shows that explicitly purport to make your child smarter.

√ Music is wonderful and does not need to be classical.

√ Avoid violence.

✓ Avoid sexy.

✓ Choose shows that you don't mind watching with your child.

✓ Avoid quizzing your child about educational shows but do talk about the shows.

How do you pick a good app or game?

Apps and games are a bit trickier. There are many apps that provide no educational value and can be exploitive. Lots of games have pop-ups that try to sell gems, treasures, and even virtual fish to young children. My younger son, Andrew, downloaded $50 worth of virtual fish for his virtual aquarium when he was 4. I learned the expensive way that your App Store settings need to be set up so the password is required for every purchase. Virtual aquarium aside, there is an endless supply of great apps for kids. Go to the Common Sense Media website for reviews before downloading. Also see the box that lists my favorite apps (as of this writing) on page 132. Other than that, here are some features to look for and features to avoid:

What to Look for in a Toddler App

✓ Easy-to-follow rules.

✓ Lots of repetition (games bordering on boring for grown-ups).

✓ Familiar toddler themes and experiences (e.g., family, animals).

✓ A design for small hands and preliterate minds.

✓ Interactive format, not too many bells and whistles.

✓ A focus on toddler milestones (e.g., nursery school, potty training).

✓ A focus on counting or colors.

✓ A focus on letters and sounds.

✓ Lots of music.

What to Avoid in a Toddler App

✓ Apps that have in-game purchases.

✓ Violence.

✓ Sexy.

✓ Advertising.

✓ Lots of bells and whistles.

✓ Games full of written text.

✓ Required keyboarding.

✓ Use of a mouse (limited use may be OK).

Be sure to set up your App Store to require your password for every purchase.

TODDLERS: BUDDING DIGITAL CITIZENS

Toddler digital citizenship is about building an ethical and empathetic foundation for your child's emerging digital experiences. These days digital citizenship is part of the curriculum, more or less officially, starting in preschool.

How do nursery schools use technology? Should I choose a nursery school based on its approach to technology?

Most important, technology at home or in school is a **tool**. Don't use a tablet because everyone else is doing it. Your toddler should use a tablet to learn her numbers or produce an interesting piece of artwork.

Right now, early childhood educators' approach to technology is all over the digital map. I suspect this is changing very quickly. There is an increasing recognition that children need to learn to use technology as a learning tool. In Manhattan private schools, the grade in which children are issued tablets gets younger every year. In 2010, my patients talked about whether they were attending a laptop high school or not. Currently, families are debating whether fourth or fifth graders are ready to take their tablets home. Technology should not replace older learning tools, but it is part of learning in the 21st century.

My Favorite Types of Apps for Toddlers

Since this is a book and not a blog, I am hesitant to list too many specific games. They are likely to be outdated before this book is published. Here, however, are some genres I recommend.

Letters/Sounds and Prereading Apps

I am not interested in apps that teach reading in this age group. Some kids read and some don't. I am more interested in engaging apps that teach letter sense and cultivate a love of reading.

- Starfall
- Grandma's Kitchen
- One More Story
- Writing Wizard

Math and Visual/Spatial Apps

- Monkey Preschool
- Tozzle
- My First Tangrams
- Elmo Loves 123s
- Little Digits
- Grover's Number Special

Creativity

- Nick Jr. Draw & Play
- Scribble Press
- My Play Home
- Faces iMake–Premium

Miscellaneous

- Everybody Has a Brain (Mac, Windows)
- Kinect Sesame Street TV (Xbox 360)

Music Apps

- Baby's Musical Hands
- Bloom HD

Some families have choice in the nursery school process and others do not. In Manhattan, you call for applications on the day after Labor Day when your child is 2 years of age. If you have a trading floor or a staff to flood the nursery schools with calls, then you may get 10 or 12 applications. It doesn't mean that you will get into any nursery schools, but you are granted the privilege of many school tours. If you live in a large city, you may have to identify the nursery schools you're interested in and get on a waitlist at conception or birth. In other places you may have a lot fewer choices or a lot less competition for spots. Whatever is the case for you, it is reasonable to ask nursery schools about their approach to technology. Have they thought about digital citizenship? How do they use technology in their classrooms? What is their opinion about toddlers and technology?

Technology has not taken over early childhood education. Early childhood educators understand the need for real play and exploration. They are coming up with innovative ways to use technology as a tool. Kids can play at virtual tangram tables where they move shapes into puzzles on a tablet. They problem-solve and build puzzles together. They can video chat or Skype with classrooms in other parts of the world.

Digital technology is also a wonderful documentation strategy. Toddlers can create audio or visual recordings of their work on an iPod Touch. They can use technology for presentations, group projects, and research. Addison's 4-year-old class did a spring unit on interviewing and reporting. They set up a TV studio in their classroom with the help of the tech department. Addison interviewed Ms. Lopez, the kindergarten teacher, and asked about her favorite flavor of ice cream and her favorite sport. The interviews were broadcast on flat screens throughout the school. At the end of the year, parents were invited for a viewing with popcorn. The 4-year-olds learned how to edit and score their documentary. They were also the anchors and reporters. They explained their findings and produced a "documentary film."

Last June, I received a flash drive with all of my daughter's artwork, school assignments, and, of course, the documentary. (This may mean that I am paying too much for nursery school, but it is cool nonetheless.) I can't honestly say that I chose Addison's school because of its approach to technology. I am very lucky to have landed in a nursery school and ongoing school with such a strong commitment to digital citizenship. However, I toured schools where they prided themselves on the number of smart boards and tablets but couldn't talk about how they taught ethical use and how it specifically enriched the academic curriculum. It was status, not substance. Other schools prided themselves on being more "traditional." They eschewed the idea of technology in the classroom prior to middle school. They explained that it was up to the parents to manage it in the early years. It is not so much about the quantity of devices but about the thoughtfulness with which the school administration approaches technology. There is a place for technology in preschool, but its use needs to be thoughtful and balanced, instilled with a sense of collaboration, creativity, and, hopefully, citizenship.

Should my toddler learn to read on digital technology?

Research is inconclusive, but Digitods (children born since 2007) need to be comfortable moving between paper and screen. Not surprisingly, parents are more engaged in print media with their toddlers but toddlers show higher levels of engagement and attention with simple e-books. The level of comprehension is the same for simple e-books and print. However, "enhanced" e-books with hyperlinks, games, and other bells and whistles detract from comprehension. Parents should not be afraid to use e-readers but should choose simple stories and not the souped-up versions that reviewers and companies often extol.[6]

I have found it to be more economical to use e-readers when your child is ready to read. Five-page picture books are cheaper online. I would still recommend using both paper books and online readers, however. Picking up a book and turning the pages does require more advanced fine-motor skills, so it can help develop those skills in your preschooler, but I don't believe that is a reason to choose paper books. Toddlers can learn these fine-motor skills throughout their daily life. I do, however, love the paper books that are truly tactile—with furry hair, sandpaper, and lift-the-flap options.

Most of the good reading apps allow you to choose narration or read mode. I always prefer that a real-life human read to a toddler. I am not sure it matters whether Mom and Dad read a virtual book from One More Story or a paper book from Barnes and Noble. Reading is one of the most important things you can do with your toddler. You model the joy of reading. You spend quality time together.

I would discourage parents from pressuring their toddlers to learn to read. The pressure creates anxiety and doesn't cultivate a love of reading and learning. Instead, I would read books with wonderful illustrations and engaging storylines. Read on whatever medium you prefer.

Older Siblings as Active Digital Citizens

Depending on who and when you ask, older siblings can be both a blessing and a curse. Recently, I ran into a friend who inquired about this book. She explained that she had just taken away technology from her 8-year-old son, Marcus, who was playing with his 4-year-old brother, Adam. Marcus was taking pictures of Adam going to the bathroom. Adam's clothes were on and they were using water to look like urine. Marcus was making videos with his smartphone, and they were both having a grand time. My friend was horrified. Her sons were not posting these videos, but she worried about how easily videos can be posted and forwarded. (We explore this topic further in chapters 9 and 10.) My friend was faced with a dilemma. She took away Marcus's phone and planned to take away technology for 2 weeks, but 2 hours later Marcus asked if he and Adam could watch a YouTube video to learn a new stitch on the Rainbow Loom. How could my friend say no? The two boys were planning to watch a video together and use it to learn the challenging "starbust" weave on the ever-popular Rainbow Loom (my current favorite toy for boys and girls ages 4–10 years).

As a part of digital citizenship, I routinely ask older siblings (like Marcus) to contribute to the family technology plan. Older siblings can help parents choose the right apps and programs. Toddlers can open icons on tablets and phones. Their ability to open an app doesn't make it appropriate for them. I would ask older siblings to help you make decisions about what is appropriate. They may understand the content better than you. By including all the family members, you are promoting a true family technology plan.

Here is an example of how to engage your older children in a discussion about the family technology plan.

JODI: Harrison, I am trying to clean up Addison's iPad. Can you help me go through all of these apps? Can you show me how to delete the apps and make some new folders?

HARRISON [AGE 9½]: Mom, that is so easy. Let me show you.

JODI: Which games do you think are appropriate for Addison [age 5½]?

HARRISON: She loves the Barbie games.

JODI: What do you think of them? Does she learn anything from them?

HARRISON: No. They are stupid, and they make you buy clothes to dress the Barbie.

JODI: Do you think that she should be buying virtual clothes for her virtual Barbie?

HARRISON: No. I don't see the point. Should we look at the games or the educational apps?

JODI: Are there any games that are also educational?

HARRISON: I like Grandma's Kitchen for her. She thinks it is a game, but she has to sound out letters and read some words. But it is fun because you bake. She also likes Monkey Math. You earn fish and mermaids for your virtual aquarium when you finish answering the questions. It is a little bit too easy for her.

JODI: What games or sites would you recommend or discourage for Addison?

HARRISON: I think that you should download the next season of *Doc McStuffins* for her. She sings along and learns about being nice to her toys and people. I am not sure that she should go on YouTube without you. She likes the kitten videos and the alphabet songs, but you never know what she might find.

JODI: Thanks for the advice. Will you let me know if you come across any games or sites that you like for her?

HARRISON: Sure, Mom. I'll check out the app store and get back to you.

TAKE-HOME POINTS

✓ You can't fight it. Technology will begin to be a part of their life.

✓ It is not too early to think about your attitudes, behavior modeling, and technology plan.

✓ Digital citizenship begins in nursery school. Older siblings can help with digital citizenship.

✓ TV/video viewing dominates most of the time your child will spend on technology.

✓ Technology is a tool for learning. It is not the end point.

✓ Toddlers are more engaged in simple e-books than print books or enhanced e-books with bells and whistles.

✓ Touch screens and apps can allow your child to develop independence and mastery.

✓ Toddler apps can stimulate early learning.

✓ Toddler TV/video programming should not substitute for real-life interaction.

✓ Toddler TV/video programming can expose your child to academic subjects.

✓ Be wary of advertising that purports to make your child smarter.

✓ There should be no TV or Internet-connected device in your child's bedroom.

✓ Parents and children need screen-free time daily.

✓ Focus for toddlers is on protecting screen-free time and using technology as a tool.

✓ Emphasis is not on total hours logged.

7 Digital Magic Years

The Calm before the Digital Storm of Middle School

Ages 6–8

About once a week, a 7-year-old boy walks into my office clutching his iPad. His mother is desperately trying to cajole him to turn it off and hand it to her. There is an unwritten rule of motherhood that you are a "bad mother" if your child can't part with his technology on demand. At this point, I ask the little boy what he has been doing on the iPad. Often, he will say that he is building something on Minecraft. That is my cue to stand up and walk over and sit next to him on the couch. I ask him to show me his Minecraft world. His mother gives the requisite groan, but he lights up as he takes me on a tour of his newest creation. This is not an isolated event. This is Minecraft.

Minecraft has over 33 million users worldwide. It is an open-ended "sand box" game that encourages creativity, resourcefulness, and patience. It is perfectly attuned to the developmental goals of 6- to 8-year-olds, who still need play yet desire independence and a sense of mastery. It is my favorite example of how 6- to 8-year-olds can use digital technology for entertainment, education, development, and independence.

Selma Freiberg's *Magic Years* is a famous account of life from the perspective of a 4- to 6-year-old child. The "magic years" have come to symbolize the awe, wonder, and fear with which young children view the world. I believe that the early elementary years are the "digital magic years." The digital world begins to open up to the young school-age child. The "control wars" have not begun yet, and there are so many quality games, apps, and websites. Children can begin to use technology independently to explore their world.

Six- to 8-year-olds have reached a number of cognitive and motor milestones that allow them to jump into much more complex, sophisticated games and apps. Their fine-motor skills allow them to use a mouse and tap away at a keyboard. Their cognitive milestones allow them to read and follow directions. They are also working so very hard at their first steps toward independence. As their interest in technology grows, they may begin to push limits and you may see the first rumblings of the inevitable "control wars."

INDEPENDENCE! INDEPENDENCE! INDEPENDENCE!: THE DEVELOPMENTAL GOALS FOR 6- TO 8-YEAR-OLDS

Independence is the mantra of the school-age child. The primary grades are a time of transition. Your children are now in school. They are no longer toddlers. First and second graders spend a lot more time in school and in activities away from home. They will be developing an identity outside of the family. They are much more aware of their social surroundings than in previous years. Their attitudes toward technology now will be shaped not only by their family but also by their peers.

Cognitive Developmental Milestones

Intellectually, 6- to 8-year-olds are becoming problem solvers. They can think about two aspects of a problem. They are able "to use their words" more, but their interactions often remain physical. Your child is in formal school, and her memory, attention span, and vocabulary are growing. She is able to think about the future and plan a little bit. However, instant gratification is the norm, and it remains difficult to wait in line and to wait until you get home to open the new toy. Your first or second grader is increasingly able to raise her hand in class and refrain from knocking everything off the kitchen table. However, impulse control is not fully developed. She can play action and shooter video games, but she is not as adroit as her older brother, because her impulse control and reaction time are slower. An old-fashioned game of Simon Says will prove my point. Your 7-year-old knows that he must follow only the directions that are preceded by "Simon says," but if he gets excited, he will be unable to inhibit the impulse to follow the command and thus he will lose the game.

Moral Developmental Goals

Kindergarten graduation classically signifies that a child can follow rules and get along well with others. First and second graders figure out what is "normal" for their family. If a 7-year-old experiences the TV on in his house all the time or endless texting at dinner, then he will normalize this as acceptable behavior. At this age, rules are very concrete. First graders have strong feelings about right and wrong, but there is no gray. Their behavior is shaped by consequences or punishment and not by internalized moral understanding. Your second-grade son, for example, will turn off the TV so his older brother can concentrate on his homework. But he is probably doing it so he won't get into trouble, not because he is a caring and empathetic brother. My 7-year-old son, Andrew, and I often talk about good and bad by using *Star Wars*-ese. The Force is good (Jedis wear white so you won't be confused), and the Dark Side is bad (Darth Vader et al. wear black). I often tell Andrew not to go toward the Dark Side. I remind him that the Force is strong inside of him. He is developing a sense of right and wrong, but his thinking remains black and white, with little room for nuance, like the epic duel between Luke Skywalker and Darth Vader.

Social and Emotional Milestones

These rudimentary, inflexible views of right and wrong enter into 6- to 8-year-olds' friendships, which become increasingly complex. Your child is developing an identity outside of her family. Your first-grade daughter will come home and be able to tell you in detail why she "hates" her best friend who accidentally spilled a juice box on her. Kids are more particular and will gravitate to friends with more similar temperaments and interests. Some children will develop strong friend-ships. Most second graders have strong opinions about whom they will play with, but parents are still making most of the social plans. Play-dates allow kids to make stronger individual connections outside of school. Parents still drive much of the socializing outside of school.

Boys and girls will play together, but single-gender groupings are becoming more and more common. Children will begin to iden-tify themselves by their interests or peers. First and second graders are increasingly capable of expressing feelings about how they look and where they fit in. They enjoy playing on teams and tolerate increased competition. Friendships are becoming increasingly important as kids spend more time away from home and begin to develop distinct inter-ests and increased ability to care about others.

Digital Milestones

How do the milestones of middle childhood impact your child's grow-ing relationship with digital technology? What is unique about this age group that matters as we create our road map for the digital era? Six- to 8-year-olds are making unique strides in the following four areas.

- Social interests
- Abiding by rules
- Literacy
- Independence

Social Interests

Peers matter in elementary school. Your children will be exposed to their peers' "norms" and family cultures. There will be children who have seen PG-13 or even R-rated movies. There will be kids with older siblings who have been exposed to more adult Internet content. There will even be a couple of kids with their own phone, maybe even a smartphone. Your early-elementary child will gravitate to friends with similar interests and temperaments. Hopefully, they will begin to be thoughtful of others and to develop an identity outside of the home. Your son's friends may begin to play Minecraft or follow basketball stats and play fantasy football. Your daughter's friends may be interested in video games, picture sharing, or watching popular YouTube videos. Whether you like it or not, your children's friends will have a strong influence over their digital interest preferences, and the development of both good and bad media habits.

Abiding by Rules

One of the hallmarks of middle childhood is the ability to follow and internalize rules. This is the moment to start thinking about rules for digital technology. This is the stage where kids figure out what is "normal." This is the moment where they can internalize the idea that thoughtful, kind, and restrained media use is the norm and not the exception. We will be formally composing a family technology plan in Chapter 12. Since parents of children this age do not report a great deal of conflict around media use, it is a perfect time to build a foundation of rules and guidelines. Permission and privilege are the first rules that your child needs to understand. Young children should ask permission to watch media and use devices. It is not a given. Digital devices are expensive, and it is a privilege, not a right, to use them.

Literacy

The code is finally broken. During middle childhood, the normally developing child learns to read. Literacy not only opens up books to children but also is a gateway to the world of digital technology. It is now possible to read websites, written text in apps, and game instructions. Increased literacy makes it easier to play more complex educational games that might explore the world of science or history. Children can now use the world of TV, computers, and the Internet to explore, create, and answer questions.

Independence is the mantra of middle childhood and is implicit to understanding all children at this age. Your child increasingly has the capability to explore digital media, devices, and the Internet on his own. He can go to YouTube and search for videos. He can navigate Club Penguin without your help. He can read reviews about different games and either read directions or figure out the directions. Increased social interaction, rule following, literacy, and independence all explain why this time period is a digital wonderland and why usage will skyrocket as your child turns 8 and 9.

MEDIA CONSUMPTION BY 6- TO 8-YEAR-OLDS

Research shows a definite increase in media usage by this age. Depending on the study, there is a 1- to 2-hour increase in usage between 5 and 6 years. At this age, usage is still heavily dependent on parents' usage, as shown in the table below. Despite school and friends, parents and family culture drive media consumption in early elementary school. (But not for long!)

Mobile devices represent the biggest change in recent years. The years 2012–2013 saw a fivefold increase in tablet ownership. Twice as many children used mobile media in 2013 as in 2011. The average amount of time that children spent on mobile devices tripled between 2011 and 2013.[1]

This is why control wars can start around this time, so it's wise to be prepared—to know what level of media usage you want your family to aim for and to put together your family tech plan to ensure that will happen.

> Most parents aren't worried about their 6-year-old's technology use, but if they don't think about it, they might end up in control wars by the time their child is 8.

Media-Related Parenting Style	Media-Centric	Media-Moderate	Media-Light
Proportion of all parents	27%	47%	26%
Parent Daily Screen Time	11 hours	4¾ hours	1¾ hours
Child Daily Screen Time	4½ hours	3 hours	1½ hours
Percent with TV in bedroom	48%	33%	28%
Percent of parents that report that TV is on whether someone is watching or not	54%	33%	19%
*Families with children ages 8 and under.			

Characteristics of families* based on media-related parenting styles.
Reprinted from Wartella et al.[2]

What do I need to know about managing technology in this age group?

■ **Use technology to explore and develop your child's interests.** In the digital magic years, technology should be used as a tool to cultivate interests and foster creativity. Your child's cognitive and motor milestones along with his striving for independence and willingness to follow rules all combine to open up a world of digital possibilities. Prior to 2007, first grade was the entry point. Although the touch-screen revolution has given kids earlier access, 6 years old still feels like the beginning in many ways. Your 6-year-old will begin to develop his or her own relationship with technology in the next 2 years. It will get solidified in middle school, but it starts now. What is exciting is that you can shape that relationship if you are involved and paying attention. First graders are amenable to rules and family guidelines, so now is the time to shape a relationship and establish a plan to avoid future conflict.

You can help shape your child's relationship with technology through your knowledge of the child's personality and temperament.

Digital technology should be a tool for cultivating interests and consequently contribute to a strong sense of self. It should help children explore and master the world around them. Children and adults use technology in different ways. The digital world can help your child explore current interests and find new ones. Is your daughter a budding fashionista or an aspiring striker? Does your son play Legos for hours, or is he a little Picasso? My son's soccer coach forwarded a link to a YouTube video showing Lionel Messi, the world's most famous professional soccer player, doing soccer drills with his teammates. If your children like sports, then download the Sports Illustrated for Kids apps. If you prefer art and fashion, then watch them create on Scribble Press or take them on a tour of Pretty Fabulous Fashion Activity, where you play, learn,

Take an interest in your child's digital life. Understand how your child uses technology.

and develop your own fashion style. The more interest you show in helping your children find worthwhile apps and games, the more likely they are to use the apps and Internet to cultivate their creativity and identity.

■ **Cultivate constructive excitement and simultaneously set down guidelines and rules.** Once the floodgates open they are difficult to close. It is a mistake to try to suppress your child's excitement. Doing so *will* start the control wars, and you'll unintentionally send an antitechnology message to your children. Technology should be viewed as a privilege, and children should ask permission to turn on the TV or get out the iPad. It should not be viewed as a carte-blanche expectation. It is not easy to be on top of the technology use, and parents are constantly "kicking themselves" for giving in on mindless games or device use in the car. Technology is so "easy" to use and so available. You should ignore writers, educators, and family members who underestimate the difficulty of setting rules around digital technology. In Chapter 12, we outline a family technology plan. The goal is to develop a flexible and reasonable approach, but no one should tell you that this is an easy task.

> Digital tech rules should be flexible and reasonable. Don't kid yourself or listen too closely to naysaying family and friends—it is not an easy task.

■ **Use technology as a tool.** I've been advocating this attitude all along, but at this age it becomes particularly important to establish that technology is not a fashion accessory or a status symbol. Technology helps you read a book, learn multiplication tables, or play a game. With enthusiasm comes the risk that your child will want the newest, latest upgrade. I prefer that first and second graders play on tablets or computers in public spaces in the home. They don't need smartphones that can be lost or taken with them (except in certain situations). At this age, I am more concerned with the quality of their usage than the quantity. Quality usage will be better on a tablet or computer where adults can play together or monitor from a distance.

> At 6–8, quality of technology usage is still more important than quantity.

■ **Emphasize quality over quantity.** Andrew, my 7-year-old son, came home with the classic second-grade neighborhood assignment. We had to explore a neighborhood in New York City and interview someone from the community. Andrew had little interest, and we kept on postponing the family field trip. Harrison (my 9-year-old son) had been working on a Keynote presentation for school (Keynote is a child-friendly PowerPoint with special effects). Andrew got excited about the fireworks that go off with each new slide and suggested that we do a Keynote presentation for his neighborhood project. After getting permission from his teacher, we set off for the Brooklyn Bridge and Grimaldi's Pizza in Brooklyn's "Dumbo" neighborhood. Armed with the iPad, we took pictures and I typed notes. Andrew spent 2 hours retyping and cropping pictures for his own slides. Each slide had special effects and musical accompaniment. We e-mailed the presentation to his teachers. The iPad did not take away from the authentic experience. We trekked over the Brooklyn Bridge and pulled on the padlocks that cover the bridge as a new symbol of everlasting love seen on bridges worldwide. We walked through puddles as we viewed the Freedom Tower from Brooklyn. We did not take a virtual tour of Brooklyn, but we used technology for documentation. The Keynote app enriched and added a new dimension to a classic elementary school assignment.

How can we use technology to make our kids smarter?

From a developmental standpoint, technology is most helpful with promoting cognitive or intellectual development in the 6- to 8-year-old age group. Sesame Workshop did a survey of apps in the iTunes App Store and Android's Google Play. They found that 80% of the apps under the heading "education" had been developed for children. Seventy-two percent of those apps aimed at children target preschool and early-elementary-age kids.

First and second graders can still learn a lot from TV. Most of the research on educational technology is related to TV. Educational TV can promote vocabulary, literacy, and basic math skills and cultivate empathy and prosocial behavior. However, the days of educational TV are numbered for your first and second graders. By third grade, they will watch TV almost entirely for entertainment, not education. Much of the educational value of TV seems to wear off once your child is fully literate. It is not that third and fourth graders can't learn a little about the world from TV, but 10-year-olds have mastered basic literacy skills and the programming changes. The programming aimed at older elementary school falls into adventure, fantasy, and soap opera genres and less into documentary and educational.

The future for your 7- and 8-year-olds is in the apps, games, and websites. There is less research on these modalities than there is on TV, so be wary of marketing. However, I would encourage your children to use educational games and play them with friends, siblings, and parents. (Specific suggestions appear near the end of this chapter.) Games can promote many aspects of cognitive and social development, such as:

- Language development
- Literacy (letter sounds, phonics, sight words)
- Writing
- Math skills and number sense
- Background information and virtual "field trips"
- Visual–spatial skills
- Problem solving
- Fine-motor skills
- Response time
- Executive planning and organization
- Creativity
- Turn taking
- Etiquette, online behavior

Literacy is obviously the hallmark academic milestone of the first and second grades. It is also important to think about math skills, storytelling, and creativity. "Joint media engagement" is the best route to getting the most out of technology at this age. The best research on reading and media, in fact, points to joint media engagement. Children gain the most from reading and playing together with parents, caregivers, and friends. They learn from discussion, questions, and the occasional teachable moments that arise. Your 7-year-old can share the experience of reading a book or playing a game with you. I would encourage you to spend time on technology with your child. You will model a healthy relationship and create teachable moments galore.

Your child may engage in technology with friends for the first time—a different type of joint media engagement. The digital world of a toddler consists largely of the phone at restaurants (and apparently on the "iPotty") and videos supervised at home. Joint media engagement with peers starts in full force in elementary school. You can restrict collaborative gaming and technology at this age if you wish. I would recommend allowing a little bit but making the distinction between interactive, collaborative play and passive, solitary play. For instance, I allow my kids to play Mario Party and Madden on the Wii for a portion of their playdates. Currently, my two boys are teaching my almost-6-year-old daughter how to race in the Wii Olympic games. They talk to each other, jump around, and play together. I do not allow Angry Birds or Temple Run on playdates. These are solitary action platform games that do not encourage interaction, dialogue, or physical activity. Kids, especially boys, will play games, but you can help your children at this age to always mix in real play and make good choices when it is time for technology.

Should I encourage my child to read e-books and use literacy apps?

Only 34% of fourth graders nationwide are reading at grade level. Literacy has become a national priority.[3] Technology must be used as a tool to aid literacy. Most of the educational apps out there are related to learning how to read. However, there are no standards, and there is limited peer-reviewed research to support the efficacy of many of the popular apps and games.

We don't really know whether e-reading is better or worse than or any different from paper reading. As I have said, I think children should read both on screens and on paper. They should be able to move fluidly between the two media. Technology does not create a love of reading. The novelty of reading a digital book wears off. Children who love to read will read on any medium. On the other hand, if your child is fascinated by technology, you can certainly use it to get him excited about reading.

I would, however, discourage kids who are learning to read from tapping on all of the links. "Enhanced" e-books and hypertext can be distracting. Studies have found in fact that it takes longer to read with hypertext, and comprehension diminishes. The ability to scan, skim, and check out links while reading is a mandatory skill for the 21st century. But it takes time to learn and should be cultivated *after* literacy is mastered.

While e-readers don't inherently make reading more fun, literacy games and apps do. There are lots of reading apps, games, and websites out there. I want to clarify here. Research supports the use of basic e-books without lots of links and games. However, games and apps that teach letters, sounds, and blends can be a great addition to your child's journey to literacy. Researchers at Sesame Workshop have referred to the education category of the App Store as "the Wild West." It is constantly changing, growing, and uncharted. Be wary of apps and games that purport to improve literacy. Some do, and some don't. As a physician, I explain to my patients that purchasing literacy and education apps is like prescribing herbal remedies. Many of them are wonderful and effective. However, the FDA does not regulate their content. Neither herbal companies nor app designers are required to provide peer-reviewed research on their efficacy. I can't guarantee the consistency of melatonin or St. John's wort over time. Parents need to be educated consumers who look at designers' credentials, read reviews, and get recommendations from respected friends and educators.

Here are some other facts from the Sesame Workshop survey of educational apps, games, and websites found on the iTunes App Store and Android's Google Play:

- 95% of e-books and games have optional narration. (Narration and subtitles are great as an option as long as they can be turned off. They give 6- to 8-year-olds the independence to read on their own but can be turned off if they are reading aloud with a grown-up.)
- 65% had embedded games and activities. (Recent research is suggesting that simpler books—more similar to print—are better for comprehension in this age group.)
- Only half of the texts offered in-text highlighting. (Digital highlighting is an important academic skill for this generation. At this age, highlighting helps kids follow along. As they get older, they will need to feel comfortable with highlighting so they can use it on digital textbooks and computerized standardized testing.)
- Most "reading apps" focus on basic skills such as letters, sounds, phonics. and word recognition. (This may be why this genre

is great for 6- to 8-year-olds. They often outgrow these games when they master literacy.)

■ Few reading apps focus on more advanced literacy skills such as comprehension and grammar. (I hope this is changing, but it explains why it is harder for older kids to find quality educational apps and games.)

■ Few apps and games list details about research or efficacy. (We are still in the Wild West here.)

■ Websites often cover a broader range of topics and offer varying grade-level curriculums. They are more likely to offer research on their effectiveness. (Websites often require a paid subscription but may offer a more sophisticated curriculum than apps.)

How can technology cultivate creativity and play?

Minecraft is the greatest invention since Lego. I rarely meet a parent who cringes when her child spends hours creating with Lego. Parents covet Legos more than children. It is common to walk into a 6- or 7-year-old's home and see Lego creations in every room. I have seen entire dining room tables covered with Star Wars Lego and family room shelves decorated with Ninjago and Chima creations.

Minecraft is even better than Lego. It can go anywhere with you and can be stored indefinitely. Minecraft can teach you about ancient Rome, city planning, art, English, and teamwork. And those are just a few examples.

A "gamemaster" on the Computer and Video Game website (CVG) summed up the brilliance of Minecraft by describing it as "an infinitely wide toybox" that generates a unique world for each person playing in single-player mode. It allows players to build progressively more sophisticated and elaborate buildings but demands that they dig around to find the best blocks, which are always stashed at the bottom of the box. After playing the game about 50 times, said this gamemaster, players will be inhabiting a bejeweled mansion, gleefully fending off spiders and zombies with custom-designed traps.[4]

Minecraft can also be played in multiplayer mode, either creative or survival. In the creative mode, players are given infinite blocks and can create, destroy, and fly without fear of "dying." Survival mode is the game mode of Minecraft. You must collect resources, manage hunger, and battle mobs. I recommend creative mode for 6- to 8-year-olds. There are no real directions, and players learn from trial and error, other players, and player-created online tutorials. (Minecraft tutorials rank high on YouTube but are not always appropriate for second graders.) Keith Stuart of *The Guardian* wrote, "It's utterly malleable. Minecraft is not a game as much as a tool." Kids feel a sense of mastery and ownership. Joel Levin, a second-grade teacher at a Manhattan private school, started MinecraftEdu with a partner from Finland. It is an international collaborative project to bring Minecraft into schools. Mojang, Minecraft's Swedish parent company, is in the process of creating discounted licenses and private servers for schools. Mr. Levin's first classroom lesson for his second graders was about online behavior. "They had to work together and show respect while playing a game just as they did in the classroom."[5]

How do I manage technology when my child goes on playdates?

Playdates are a staple of nursery and elementary school children's lives. There is a shift in the first grade to the dreaded or beloved dropoff playdate. Parents and caregivers of young children spend a great deal of time at playdates. Often nursery school children engage in parallel play while their parents or caregivers engage in more reciprocal interactions. The good news about 4-year-old playdates is that family rules can be taken along with you. It was always clear to me which parents could tolerate the Nerf guns or the Wii Olympics. This all changes with the dropoff playdate or sleepover. Do you know what your kids are doing on these playdates? Your kids will be influenced by their friends. Certainly, if the playdate is held at a home with older children your child might be exposed to inappropriate media.

At my home, we try to limit media on playdates but don't completely ban it. I don't mind the kids playing on the Wii with each other since I know the games and they are generally interactive. However, I encourage more time off media than on it. Kids should not go on the Internet during a playdate unless supervised by an adult. I will let my children watch a Rainbow Loom video on YouTube, but I want an adult to restrict or co-view other videos. In general, I discourage passive TV during playdates. Sometimes if the kids are exhausted or there has been lots of fighting or expressed emotion, then TV can create some quiet, wind-down time. Your kids should view playdates as a time to hang out, run around, talk, and play.

I can't control what goes on at other homes, and neither can you. If you have a relationship with the family, you can ask about Internet, games, and TV. In general, it is time to be clear with your kids about your rules. They may not always follow them, but it is worth a try to be clear. I would avoid telling your 7-year-old daughter that she can't use any technology on playdates unless you have clearly stated this to the other family, which is probably unrealistic. I would take a more flexible approach; some ways you might phrase your thoughts to your child are in the box on page 153.

> You can't control technology use at someone else's home, but you can convey clear expectations to a 6- to 8-year-old.

Do I need to worry about social media at this point?

Yes and no. Parents of 6- to 8-year-olds are not worried about social media. Most Internet use is still parentally controlled. YouTube offers the biggest risk at this age. There is so much wonderful stuff to watch, but it takes only one click—or less—to find widely popular but inappropriate material. At this age, children should not have YouTube accounts and should never post videos on YouTube. YouTube can be a wonderful opportunity for joint media engagement. Children can truly enjoy it and find videos that are relevant to their lives. My children's first exposure to YouTube was the song "When Two Vowels Go Walking" from PBS's *Between the Lions*, with its refrain "When two vowels go walking, the first one does the talking" (i.e., when two vowels appear next to each other, you pronounce only the first vowel sound). This vowel song has almost 1 million viewers and has allowed for hilarious joint media engagement.

> YouTube offers great joint media engagement opportunities, but kids should not have YouTube accounts and should never post videos on YouTube.

How to Tell Your 6- to 8-Year-Old
How to Manage Technology Use on a Playdate

"We don't use technology during playdates at our home, but other families have different rules."

"You are a big girl/boy and you will have to make good decisions at your friend's house."

"You can tell your friend that you would prefer to play a real board game or outside game instead of the Wii, DS, or iPad."

"You can tell your friend that you are not allowed to watch grown-up TV or movies, but you are allowed to watch Nick, PBS, or Disney Jr."

"If you want to play a video game with a friend for a while, then you might suggest playing a real game first and ending the playdate with the iPad or the Xbox."

"If your friend insists on playing video games, then do your best to be supportive and respectful while playing. If the game gets out of hand or there is a lot of bad language, you can tell your friend that you are feeling uncomfortable with this game and could we try another one or turn it off altogether."

"Try to choose games (both real and virtual) where you can really interact or play with your friend. Examples of good video games might be Dance Party Karaoke and Wii/Xbox sports games."

"Try to choose games where you are taking turns and talking to each other. Try not to play games where you will sit next to each other and not talk."

"I do not want you on the Internet or Instagram when you are at a friend's house unless supervised by a grown-up (not an older brother or sister)."

"You will not get in trouble for your technology use on a playdate, but I would like you to be honest with me about what you did."

Parents should also be aware of multiplayer games and child-friendly social network forums—"SNFs" or "social looping" sites. Many games have single- and multiplayer modes. For example, I would discourage 6- and 7-year-olds from playing Minecraft on the multiplayer mode. Minecraft is a developmentally appropriate game in the single-player mode. However, you might allow your kids to play apps and games against friends whom you know and not allow kids of this age to play against strangers.

There are social networking sites that are geared toward 6- to 12-year-olds. Disney's Club Penguin is a hugely popular virtual world for elementary school kids. The site gets millions of visits per month. Children create penguin avatars and can chat and play with friends in a cartoon environment. You can decorate your igloo and care for your puffle. Paid membership brings many more opportunities to dress and decorate. Kids can encounter mean behavior, but there are lots of parental controls. Children can earn virtual coins for charity, and there is an online newspaper to promote good citizenship. I would encourage

---

 Sources of Digital Product Reviews

- **Common Sense Media:** Common Sense Media is the best place to look up movies, videos, games, or apps that your children ask about. The reviews are developmentally appropriate and helpful.
- **Parents' Choice Awards:** Since 1978, the Parents' Choice Foundation has been giving awards to toys and media for children. I trust them and would consider any of their award-winning games, software, or apps.
- **Yogiplay:** Yogiplay sends you app recommendations customized for your children's age and gender.
- **Children's Technology Review:** Subscription review that provides "consumer reports" on interactive media products. Ad-free and has been around since 1993.
- **Kindertown:** Offers reviews and suggestions. App developers submit their games, and Kindertown reviews only games and apps that they deem educational.

you to initially use this site with your child as an opportunity to teach about safety, etiquette, and time management.

Some Questions You Might Ask Your Child about Social Media

✓ "How long do you think you should spend on Club Penguin?"

✓ "Can you show me your avatar, igloo [Club Penguin], or new structure?"

✓ "Can you show me an example of someone not being nice on the site?"

✓ "Are there rules for this site? What are they?"

✓ "Can you show me or tell me an example of someone not following the rules?"

✓ "What do you like best about this site?"

✓ "Have you been asked to buy anything on this site? Are there in-app purchases?"

✓ "Would you recommend this site or game to your friends? Why? Why not?"

Is my child old enough for a flip phone or a smartphone?

No. But there are some exceptions. As we all know, phones are not created equal. Most middle schoolers differentiate between a "flip phone" (old-school cellular phone) and a smartphone (phone that connects to the Internet). I can't think of any reason to give a first or second grader a smartphone, but there may be a reason for a flip phone. The decision to give your child a phone is a very personal family choice. As a general rule, it is time for a phone when a child is consistently dropped off by himself or traveling by himself. I have not observed a great deal of phone pressure at this age, but the discussion has usually begun. Ask your second grader if anyone in her class has a phone. She will likely be able to tell you the names and brands of any phone owners. She may also tell you who is expecting a phone for Christmas or a birthday.

Reasons for Giving a Flip Phone at This Age

✓ Parents are divorced and the child would like to have more control over his or her communication with the other parent.

✓ Parents are divorced and there is shuttling back and forth. Communication may be helpful and may ease the transition between two homes.

✓ A child is taking long school bus rides and needs to communicate with parents for some reason.

✓ The child has a chronic medical condition and needs a phone in case there is an urgent need to reach the parents.

✓ The child has a chronic medical or psychiatric condition and misses a lot of school and can benefit from a phone to stay in touch with friends.

Otherwise, there is no good reason to give a child a cellphone. I tried to give my son Harrison a flip phone when he was 7 years old. It was a developmental disaster.

The sports van had dropped him off at our home after a game. The driver didn't wait for us to come get him, and he was left with a friend on the street. They walked to the friend's apartment building on the corner. They didn't have to cross any streets or deal with strangers, but I was beside myself. The next day, I bought him a phone. He put it in his backpack and never looked at it again. Presumably, it ran out of charge and got stuck at the bottom of his backpack with the papers, Gummy Bears, and Pokémon cards.

> The decision to buy a phone should be well thought out by all parents.

Eventually, I realized that it was useless and that he didn't need a phone. We picked him up from school and took him to activities. He was almost always with an adult. I gave the phone to my assistant, and it took my son 6 weeks to realize that I had repossessed it. I recognize that other children may have responded differently at this age. But he wasn't ready, and I had bought it out of fear and anxiety. More to come on this topic as your child grows up.

How do I choose good apps and games for my children?

Use reviews and recommendations. Encourage educational games and apps. Ask your children to walk you through any games they want you to purchase. Try to play together the first time so you have a good sense of the pros and cons.

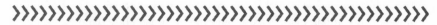

Guidelines and Recommendations for 6- to 8-Year-Olds

Reading and Literacy

Websites may be better for literacy than apps.

Online Reading

- **One Minute Reader:** Leveled apps that focus on reading fluently. Child reads short passages aloud with narrator and then reads on her own for fluency and accuracy.
- **Raz Reader:** Expensive but amazing grouping of e-books with narration option and short comprehension quizzes.
- **Laz Reader:** Laz Reader e-books are bought on the App Store through a company called Learning A–Z. They provide basic leveled books at a lower cost and without the bells and whistles.
- **Story Before Bed:** Allows for prerecorded narration so you can read a story to your child when you are away.
- **Speakaboo:** E-reading website with lots of classic books in e-version.
- **Oceanhouse Media:**
  - Website and publishers of educational apps that "uplift, educate and inspire."
  - Develop e-books and games around children's classics such as Berenstain Bears and Dr. Seuss.

Reading Apps/Games

- **Starfall:** One of the best apps out there for learning letters and sounds.
- **PBS Ready to Learn:**
  - PBS's initiative to teach reading.
  - Includes apps, games, and shows like *Super Why.*
- **Cosmos Chaos:** An example of a video-game-style app designed to increase your child's vocabulary.

Math

Worthwhile Apps and Websites

- **IXL:** Websites that help kids meet the standards of the Common Core. They offer exercise and interactive games for math and language arts for grades K–12. It can be expensive but offers a broad curriculum and sends reports to parents about children's progress.
- **Splash Math:** A website with multiple math apps that can be used on multiple platforms and is appropriate for grades K–5. The goal is to turn mundane worksheets into interactive games.
- **AB Math:** Site that has several downloadable math apps.
- **Brownie Points:** Parents purchase Common Core math workbooks, and children are rewarded with games like Angry Birds when they complete each module.
- **Math Ninja:** Free app where you use your math skills to defend your tree house against Hungry Tomato and his robotic army.
- **Save the Sushi:** Evil Queen has stolen the Golden Sushi. Use your multiplication skills to recover it. Better for 8+.

Creativity

Encourage any game that cultivates creativity.

- **Minecraft:** See description on page 138.
- **Toontastic:**
  - Create your own cartoon.
  - Record your own stories and then animate them.
- **Doodlecast:**
  - Creative presentations on the iPad.
  - Draw pictures or use photos.
  - You record your story and doodle on the image and create your own videos.
- **Out-A-Bout:** Use real photos to tell stories.

Physical Activity

Encourage console games with physical activity and interactions.

- **Wii Party U:** Old-fashioned family games that teach teamwork and encourage family time.

- **New Super Mario Bros:** Traditional platform games that encourage lots of teamwork.
- **Kinect:** Motion sensors for the Xbox consoles that allow players to move and interact with the games.

Social Network Starters

- **Club Penguin:** A massive multiplayer game where penguins are the avatars and there is a virtual world of igloos, games, and puffles.
- **iTwixie:**
  - A social media site for girls from 7 to 12 years of age.
  - Girls can create their own blogs, vote on favorite books, or take the vocabulary word of the week challenge.
  - Girls can chat with other girls from around the world and all communication is monitored by iTwixAdmin.

Caution

- Be wary of in-app purchases.
- Better to download paid apps without advertising and in-app purchases.
- Be aware of multiplayer games:
  - Choose single-player modes.
  - Play only against parent-approved friends in multiplayer mode.

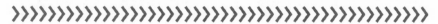

TAKE-HOME POINTS

✓ Technology should be viewed as a tool.

✓ Technology should be used to cultivate your child's interests.

✓ Technology will begin to be used socially at this age.

✓ Technology should encourage mastery and independence.

✓ Technology should be treated with respect and require permission for use.

✓ At this age, kids will begin to have their own relationship with the digital world.

✓ Go online with your child ("joint media engagement").

✓ Developmentally, this is a great time to create rules.

✓ YouTube requires parental involvement.

✓ Technology should be used to promote literacy and the joy of reading.

✓ I love Minecraft (in moderation, of course).

✓ Role play with your child prior to drop-off playdates/sleepovers.

✓ Encourage exploration and honesty.

✓ Be aware of ads and in-app purchases.

✓ There is less educational TV programming at this age.

✓ There are lots of educational games and apps for this age.

✓ Your child is probably not ready for a phone yet. There are exceptions.

✓ You can choose to introduce social media or not, but it is available.

8 Welcome to the Frequent Flyer Club

Equipped with a Digital Boarding Pass and Ready to Take Off

Ages 8–10

My husband and I had dinner with friends who have 5- and 10-year-old boys. They were telling us about having recently toured kindergartens for their younger son. They had visited a very highly esteemed all-boys' school and were surprised at the school's approach to technology. The school felt it was important to protect the kids, and technology wasn't formally introduced until sixth grade. Kids were told not to use Google in the lower school. This couple considered themselves "old school," but this seemed extreme to them. My friend actually walked out of the school, withdrew her application, and bought two iPads for the boys for Christmas. Her husband laughed and said, "We bought iPads, but we aren't letting them use them. We have decided to eliminate all technology during the week."

I was surprised. This proclamation seemed a bit draconian for a couple who prided themselves on being flexible and reasonable and on not imposing lots of hard-and-fast rules—despite describing themselves as "old school." The husband explained that they had been at the fourth-grade cocktail party the night before, where the parents were all buzzing about a group of boys who were up at 4:00 A.M. playing Clash of Clans. My friends had been told that their very rule-abiding son was part of the group. They went home and asked their soft-spoken son if he was up at four in the morning playing games. He was shocked and angry. He said that he was certainly not up at 4:00 A.M. playing games.

How could they accuse him of waking up at 4:00 A.M. to play games?! He set his alarm for *5:00* A.M. to play Clash of Clans.

It has started. You are on the slippery slope to losing control of technology in your family. Parents with children under age 8 don't worry about technology. It doesn't even make their top 10 list of general life concerns.[1] Concerns change, however, at around age 8 and the end of elementary school. Usage skyrockets! Where your son or daughter used technology (on average) for 2–4 hours per day between ages 6 and 8, you might expect usage to jump to 6–8 hours by age 10.

I start this chapter with 8-year-olds even though we covered age 8 in the preceding chapter because this seems to be the swing year. Researchers study kids 8 and under and kids 8–18 years of age. At 8, kids begin to have their own relationship with technology. They may begin to use technology in school, and their friends will have preferences and may be tablet and smartphone owners. They are developing their own relationship with digital technology. Obviously, their use of digital media is still dictated by parental control, but the connection between parental usage and child usage is becoming unhinged. And the issues are becoming more numerous and more complex, as you'll see in this chapter. Now social media has entered your child's universe and technology will shape his or her identity further. Your child has become eligible for true digital citizenship—more freedom, more decision making, and more responsibility.

> Age 8 is a swing year for technology use.

IDENTITY, DIGITAL CITIZENSHIP, AND SOCIAL FOCUS: DEVELOPMENTAL GOALS IN THE LATE ELEMENTARY YEARS

Milestones that are particularly relevant to digital usage at this age are shown in the box on page 164.

Cognitive Milestones

Academically, school is ramping up. They are no longer learning to read but reading to learn. Children may experience academic stress and challenges for the first time. They will begin to shape their identity based on their success at school. Your kids are reading chapter books and writing stories, and the math is getting more complicated. They are beginning to converse and relate more like adults. You may be seeing the first signs of abstract thinking. However, your child will quickly revert to concrete thinking when stressed. Third and fourth graders have an increased attention span and will begin to prepare for middle school.

Physical Milestones

Physically, your third and fourth graders are beginning to show the earliest signs of puberty, especially girls. Kids become more aware of physical gender differences. Muscles are more well developed, and kids at this age can handle athletics that demand endurance. Their fine-motor advances lead to better handwriting and more sophisticated art-work. Kids will generally become expert "keyboarders," partly due to increased fine-motor skills and an increased desire to use computers independently.

Since digital technology usage skyrockets, parents need to be care-ful to protect their child's sleep and exercise. Some kids may choose sedentary television viewing over more physical activities. Kids also need their sleep to grow, stay healthy, and manage their increasingly demanding days. Kids are on the heels of puberty, and physical changes are a huge part of their life.

Social, Emotional, and Moral Development

Eight- to 10-year-olds are developing their own moral compass. They have a growing sense of empathy and can begin to understand oth-ers' point of view. They are broadening their understanding of right and wrong. I wouldn't classify them as morally sophisticated, but they are a step beyond the *Star Wars* "Force" and "Dark Side" black-and-white moral thinking that we saw so vividly in early elementary. They can recognize acts of kindness and internalize respect. They can increasingly identify kind versus bullying behavior online. They have increased ability to respect and care for their devices.

Developmental Milestones That Are Critical to Digital Technology Use

- Usage skyrockets!!!
- Empathy develops.
- Gender roles and stereotypes are internalized.
- Empathy and a more finely tuned moral compass enable kids to identify disrespectful behavior, online as well as off.
- Increased abstract thinking allows for more complex games and use of computers.
- Kids this age can internalize and understand the need for safety.
- Increase in responsibility and cognitive abilities has led many schools to introduce tablets and computers into fourth grade.

Emotionally, kids are developing a stronger sense of identity. Friendships are more complex and more likely to be single gender. Nine- and 10-year-olds will vehemently deny interest in the opposite sex, but increased teasing and flirting is evident. Parents should monitor picture-sharing sites like Snapchat because there is increased risk of inappropriate pictures and comments being exchanged. Gender patterns in media use emerge. We see that boys will increasingly play video games together while girls will opt out of console games. Girls will continue to play games on their portable devices and will increasingly communicate via pictures and texts. Peer pressure is rearing its ugly head. Kids will become very aware of and vulnerable to peer pressure if they lack self-confidence.

The convergence of all the development that 8- to 10-year-olds experience opens a lot of new digital doors for them. Increasingly, kids will use technology for school. Educators recognize how technology can aid in developing abstract thinking. The fact that kids this age are also capable of more complex thinking means that many games and apps intended to be entertaining can also have high educational value.

The leaps they are making in social, emotional, and moral development also carve out a different digital landscape: Kids will begin to communicate via social networking, e-mails, and texts for the first time. Online misbehavior and the first elements of cyberbullying may emerge. Differentiation in gender roles exposes kids to violence via video games (mainly boys) and to negative body image and stereotypes (mainly girls). At this stage it's crucial to translate home values and mores to your child's technological environment. You have the opportunity to teach right and wrong as well as respect and etiquette using technology. Some applications and suggestions appear later in this chapter.

I'll also talk more about rules. The rules need to crystallize so your expectations are clear, but your parenting and discipline have to evolve too. At this age kids need to understand their mistakes and the reasons for discipline and rules. They will need to take their family rules and values out into the world. They do much better when their parents explain the reasons for certain decisions and limits.

Fourth graders are able to set goals for themselves. They can reflect on their own interests and seek to gain new skills. Kids' relationship with technology will become more apparent as their identity emerges through these media.

Late elementary is the transition from being a "little kid" to being a middle school tween. Most kids are eager to be seen as "big kids" and to take on new responsibilities and roles. Pre-tweens need to understand the logic behind family rules and boundaries, but they may also start to push back with their parents if they find the rules to be unreasonable.

SKILLED NAVIGATION: TECHNOLOGY USAGE IN LATE ELEMENTARY SCHOOL

As noted above, kids ages 8–10 spend 6–8 hours per day on digital media. This does not include homework or time spent talking and texting on a cell phone. The usage time only increases from age 8 to 18 years in every platform except video games, which peaks prior to age 15. The combination of extra time with technology and developmental readiness for new tools, like smartphones, makes this age group eager to participate. At this stage, we see that children's usage is not as closely aligned to parents' usage. Since kids will be on digital media all the time, the rules need to be codified and parents will gain lots of practice enforcing them.

Technology usage seems to be highest when there's a TV in the bedroom, TV is often on in the background, and no media rules are in place.

A 2010 Kaiser Family Foundation study showed that access to TV and the presence or absence of media usage rules had a significant effect on children's usage at this age. TV in the bedroom, background TV, and media rules are the three factors that seem to affect usage the most. As shown in the bar graph below, kids with no bedroom TV, no background TV, and at least some rules have significantly lower usage.[2]

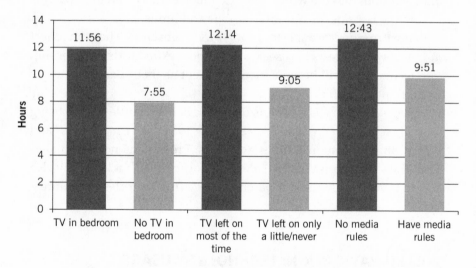

Media exposure among 8- to 18-year-olds by TV environment and rules. Adapted from Rideout et al.[3]

Other shifts to be aware of:

■ Approximately 31% of 8- to 10-year-olds own cell phones.
■ Boys are exposed to approximately 1 hour more of media time per day, which comes from use of video games.
■ 20% of 8- to 10-year-olds use social networking on a regular basis.

These numbers represent a significant shift in how kids actually use technology. Most 6- to 8-year-olds use a cell phone only when handed a parent's phone to play a game while out to dinner with parents; by ages 8–10 almost a third of them actually own one. Social networking was not part of their daily activity, unless they were looking over the shoulder of older siblings, but now one in five is a regular visitor to Instagram and other social platforms.

NAVIGATING THE CROSSROADS: DIGITAL TECHNOLOGY AT A MAJOR DEVELOPMENTAL TRANSITION

There's a lot to think about once your child reaches age 8. As a reminder of what you should consider and plan for, see the box on page 168. In the following pages I've answered the questions parents ask most often in each of these four areas.

Rules

Should I limit all technology?

"Moderation, moderation" is the name of the parenting game. I have two parenting analogies for moderation parenting. If you have ever attended a kindergarten or first-grade birthday party, you will be able to observe the candy obsession. There is always one child who devours the cake, the ice cream, and the candy. Often this is a child who is not allowed sweets or treats at home, but placed in a social setting where parents can't interfere, the child jumps straight into the chocolate cake. Jump forward 12 years, to the teenager who has to sneak out in the middle of the night and the college freshman who is drunk the entire year. Often these young adults will head to extreme behavior because they felt that their parents were too strict. They didn't learn how to manage food, alcohol, or partying when they were at home. You can sniff these kids out in the digital world as well. They run to the forbidden iPad or video game. They are obsessed

> Don't restrict technology; learn to use it wisely.

Digital and Developmental Milestones for 8- to 10-Year-Olds

1. **RULES: Your child now has the ability to understand and internalize family and social rules.**
   - Technology limits
   - Need for parental controls
   - Need to take family rules with you at sleepovers and camps

2. **IDENTITY: Your child is rapidly developing an identity and distinct personality.**
   - Digital citizenship and digital footprint
   - Use of technology to aid in identity development
   - Etiquette and respect online and offline
   - Seeds of bullying and cyberbullying

3. **INDEPENDENCE AND INDEPENDENT FRIENDSHIPS: Increasingly your child will socialize without you in the middle.**
   - World of social networking
   - Instagram
   - Flip phones and smartphones

4. **SEXUALITY AND BODY IMAGE: Your child will become aware of societal expectations and her body.**
   - Emerging gender roles
   - Body image
   - Birds and the bees

with deceiving their parents. The take-home message is that kids need to learn how to manage and live with technology, which means they need access.

What types of rules should I have?

- Keep technology out of the bedroom as much as possible.
- Don't let your kids sleep with technology.
- Teach your children to ask permission to use technology.
- Limit weekday technology (this will vary from family to family).

- Download/buy games and apps yourself, don't let your children do so.
- Oversee YouTube.
- Keep family computers in as public a space as possible.
- Tell your children to report inappropriate games/sites/social networks to you.
- Don't permit technology use during meals.
- Designate screen-free times for the entire family.
- Make technology a privilege, not a right.

Developmentally, your kids are able to follow rules but are much more likely to abide by and internalize rules that they fully understand. I recommend calling a family meeting and asking all family members to contribute a rule to the list. This meeting can be a forum for explaining the rationale of all rules agreed on. Don't forget to make rules for yourself too and ask your kids to help enforce them.

A very respected colleague of mine explained her family's "spanking rule" to me. Don't get the wrong idea. She and her husband have three beautiful daughters ages 7, 9, and 11, and they don't believe in spanking their children. However, the parents agreed (in a playful way) to allow the girls to "spank" the parents if the parents used their phones at inappropriate times such as at dinner, while driving, or during family time. My friend acknowledges being chained to her phone, texts, and e-mails 24/7. Her daughters' humorous "spanking" reminds her that she needs to keep her technology use in check.

What about tablets and portable video game players in the bedroom?

When my son Harrison was 8, he had his first sleepover with a 9-year-old friend. Dylan was lovely and polite but had a lot of trouble falling asleep. He convinced Harrison that he needed his iPad to fall asleep, so Harrison snuck downstairs and secured it for him. When they woke up the next morning, Andrew, my middle child (who was 6 at the time), explained that Dylan really needed his iPad because it was like Andrew's "blankie," which he slept with nightly. Kids (and adults) sleep with their devices. Dylan was a heavy media user, and I truly believe that he felt more comfortable falling asleep in a strange place hugging his iPad. Technology has become an appendage or an "iBlankie" for many of us.

I highly recommend that your kids have alarm clocks. I would discourage kids from using their computers, tablets, or phones as alarm clocks. Doing so fosters a sleep association that we want to discourage or, better yet, never start. There is a plethora of research showing that bedroom TV leads to less physical activity, obesity, lower grades, and so forth. The research isn't complete on computers, tablets, phones, and Internet in the bedroom. It is clear to me that computers and Internet access in the bedroom can lead to poor sleep and problematic, unsupervised usage.

> Technological devices should not be the last thing you touch before bed and the first thing you think about when you wake up.

I encourage all of my elementary school students to do homework in a public space. Ironically, this reduces distraction. It also makes it easier to get help when needed. I have found that kids are less likely to get on the Internet or fall asleep when reading and studying if they are out of their bedrooms. This applies to digital technology as well. It is unrealistic to recommend that kids be monitored all the time or that adults use technology with their children all the time. However, it is less likely that the e-book will turn into Angry Birds if there is a chance that a grown-up will walk by and notice.

Are parental controls, timers, and child-friendly tablets helpful?

The first time I had difficulty getting my 9-year-old off his iPad, my 7-year-old said, "Mom, you should have bought him a Nabi 2." He was referring to Fuhu's line of Nabi tablets designed for kids that come with built-in timers. Was he right? Should I buy only devices with timers? Should I install Net Nanny or MamaBear, two of the most popular parental control systems? I didn't love the "big brother" approach to managing technology, so these weren't easy questions to answer.

Developmentally, executive functioning is the last part of the brain to develop. Executive planning allows you to inhibit risky behavior and think before you act. It allows you to think about the consequences and plan long term. Kids need their parents to manage planning and consequences at this time. Most adults I know (myself included) have trouble managing their time on their devices. Timers and clear time limits can help kids manage their time. Parental monitoring and involvement can help kids think about the consequences of their online actions.

I do believe in timers and time limits on devices. Kids should know how much time they have and should be able to get off the device when the time is up. Whether to buy devices that do the work for you is a personal choice. I am hoping that in the future most devices marketed for both adults and kids will have built-in turn-off timers. Off Remote is an app that allows you to remotely turn off computers. You can turn off the computer that your child is playing on if needed. There is an entire industry involved in getting your child off his computer. Kidoff software can be installed on the computer that your child uses. You will be able to talk to your child's computer from another computer via your home network. You can send text and audible reminders and shut down their computers if needed. It reminds me of a fire drill. It is practice for when they will be able to turn their devices off on their own. Nabi, Kurio, and Kindle Fire all market internal timers for kids. I choose to use an old-school kitchen timer to help my family set time limits.

Parental controls are slightly different. In general, I don't recommend them because the goal is to have family rules and set limits that ultimately will be internalized and adhered to by each individual. The goal is to trust your kids and check in periodically. Parental controls like Net Nanny and WebWatcher are sophisticated filtering systems that can block and track your children. They can provide the content of e-mails and messages, and they can show Facebook activity for 24 hours. Some will notify you each time your child posts on Instagram. With the MamaBear app, parents download the app onto their phones and set it up with their family. Kids install and log in to MamaBear. Kids can check in with emoticons or send "come get me" alerts. Parents can monitor location, driving, and components of social media. Most 8- to 10-year-olds don't need MamaBear yet, but they do need help setting timers and limits and using their devices safely.

How do I manage technology on sleepovers?

I spoke at length about drop-off playdates in the last chapter, where you'll find suggestions for starting a discussion on the topic. Your child will have greater freedom at this point, and technology is less likely to be monitored on playdates and sleepovers. With third and fourth graders, I recommend telling the host family what devices you are sending along, such as the iPhone or DS or games for the Wii. The host parents can help your child care for this expensive equipment and increase the chances that it returns home. More important, giving them this information opens the door for a brief discussion.

Your child will know whether technology will be a primary component of a sleepover. At this age, children are very in tune with who has which devices and who is a "gamer" or who is "always on Instagram" and who is not. Of course, if the friend has older siblings, then the household is more likely to have more devices and more mature games and movies. You don't have control when you send your child on a sleepover, but you have more control when you host one. You can model good technology behavior when your child has sleepovers. A model dialogue appears below.

How to Talk to Kids at a Sleepover at Your Home

MOM: Welcome to our place. What are you all planning on doing tonight?

YOUR CHILD: We are going to play Mario Party for a while, and I want to show Michael that hilarious kitten video on YouTube, and then we are going to watch the Knicks play the Thunder.

MOM: Michael, what would you like to do? Does your mom let you play on the Wii? YouTube?

MICHAEL: My mom says it's OK to play on the Wii, but she doesn't want me on the Internet. I am not really into basketball.

MOM: Son, why don't you play the Wii for half an hour, and then I will help you two find a board game to play. Let's try to find a sports game or movie that Michael is interested in and his parents will approve of.

I have found that it is easy to default to tablets and console games on playdates. You may need to brainstorm with your kids prior to sleepovers about alternatives to media use. It will require more work on your part but will result in sleepovers that are more balanced and interactive.

Identity Development

Should I be concerned about my child's digital footprint?

As discussed in Chapter 1, you probably need to be concerned about your child's digital footprint when you post your baby's first bath photo. California law SB 568, which has been dubbed the "online eraser" law, was enacted in 2013 and will go into effect in 2015. The law allows minors to erase posts and pictures. It is a well-intentioned law, but none of us really believe that anything online is "erasable." The NSA is capable of storing and retrieving our e-mail messages, so I assume that everything is retrievable.

Parents control most of the footprint up until the end of elementary school. In this age group I recommend focusing on digital citizenship more than footprint. We are trying to build a safe, kind, and ethical foundation for your child's digital life. Developmentally, your children are old enough to grasp the concept of a digital footprint. They may not fully understand what "forever" means or the consequences of drunken high school pictures for college admissions. We don't want to frighten our kids, but they are capable of understanding that a footprint is a reflection of their real and digital selves. We want them to post their artwork, poems, and opinions. We want them to become good digital citizens.

Common Sense Media offers a great lesson plan for introducing digital citizenship. It is entitled Super Digital Citizen. The lesson starts with an explanation of Spider-Man's motto: "With Great Power Comes Great Responsibility." Children are asked to define digital citizenship and create a digital superhero and comic strip where the hero "saves the day."[4] The digital super hero may stop online rumors, challenge mean words, or prevent password sharing. A digital citizen is more than someone who uses the Internet. It is someone who is safe, responsible, and respectful.

How can technology cultivate identity development?

If you've read this book from the beginning, you've already heard my tirades on the fact that technology is a tool. Here I go again. By age 8, kids are developing unique personalities and interests. Digital technology can help them explore and embrace their online and offline interests. My children's school uses the acronym ACE to explain its approach to technology. ACE stands for *apply, create, explore.*

When Harrison turned 9, he began to have an independent relationship with technology. He started taking "tech" at school, and his friends use technology in all kinds of ways. He started with fantasy football. He drafted a team that he follows on his fantasy football app. He e-mails his friends (and their dads) when he wants to make trades. His 9-year-old cousin introduced him to Math Brownie Points. It is an app where you pay for a math module but the kids receive "brownie points" as they progress through each module. When they complete the module, they "win" a choice of game apps. Harrison "won" Angry Birds–Star Wars edition.

At school he was introduced to Keynote, which is a kids' version of PowerPoint. I returned from an out-of-town medical conference, and he greeted me with a Keynote welcome-home presentation that included fireworks and special effects (I especially enjoyed this app).

Harrison has also begun to learn Garage Band. He is actually making music. He makes up lyrics, which he "yells" into the iPad (he thinks that real rock singers "yell"), mixes his voice with the music, and creates a dance party mix for his brother and sister.

Harrison's friend Zoe uses technology to decorate cakes, create nail designs, and work on her Spanish homework. Two girls in Harrison's class are writing a book together on Google Docs. When I meet kids in my office or my life, I often ask them what they like to do online. I end up learning a great deal about who they are or who they want to become. Often, I will share my patients' online interests with their parents. Parents are often surprised that I learned so much about their kids by better understanding their online interests.

Take a genuine interest in your child's digital interests. When possible, try playing a game with your 9-year-old. See if you can beat his Flappy Bird score or remember more state capitals in Stack the States.

Ask your child for a tour of his Minecraft masterpieces or Club Penguin igloos. By taking an interest, you are creating an atmosphere of openness. You can monitor safety and appropriate behavior, but you want to keep an open dialogue. You want your children to feel that you have a genuine interest in their activities. It should not be about spying but rather about sharing.

Should I worry about cyberbullying?

All children and teenagers using social networking, e-mail, or texts are at risk for cyberbullying. However, in third and fourth grade, the goal is to teach responsible use. My children's school teaches technology in conjunction with its ethics curriculum. The elementary and middle school ethics curriculum is built around self, others, and surroundings (SOS). Kids are taught to be mindful of themselves, their friends, and their community online. They are given iPads in fourth grade but not allowed to take them home. The goal is to be responsible and respectful of technology and have the cognitive skills to fully utilize the technology independently by age 10. The school wants them also to learn empathy for their classmates and community before they are allowed to be online independently in fifth grade.

Learning online etiquette and kindness is not simple. I encourage parents to help kids with their first texts, posts, and pictures. It takes experience to learn how to post pictures responsibly. I ask 9- and 10-year-olds to think before they post and to ask themselves a few simple questions:

"Would I be OK if someone else posted a similar picture of me?"

"Is this a picture or text that I would want my grandparents to see?"

"Is there anything embarrassing or weird about this post/picture?"

"Is there any chance that I could hurt anyone's feelings with this post/picture?"

I have a 10-year-old patient who posted a picture of a friend picking his nose. Another friend commented that the picture was wrong and should be taken down. My patient was devastated and cried in my office. He never meant to hurt anyone's feelings. He hadn't taken the picture. He reposted it and thought it was funny. Initially, it was difficult for him to understand how it might be seen as inappropriate.

Kids who are 8–10 years old are beginning to understand empathy, but it is not yet fully developed. My patient understood that "picking your nose" was embarrassing but didn't realize that his friend might be uncomfortable with him posting the picture. It was just a step beyond the funny and gross stuff that 9-year-old boys like. This is a mild but realistic example. The only way that kids will learn about respect and kindness online is to be part of an ongoing dialogue and be able to post, make mistakes, and grow from them.

Social Networks and Independence

Your third and fourth graders will experience their first social contact online if they have not done so already. E-mails, texts, multiplayer games, and Instagram are the introduction to social networks. Some kids are ready for the pressures of social networking, and others are not. The head of elementary technology at one Manhattan school told me that she often hears fourth and fifth graders talking about the stress of texts. Some kids will stop texting because the barrage of incoming messages becomes onerous and tiring. There are misunderstandings and too much responsibility.

Since 9- and 10-year-olds are developing media independence, we should arm them with safety rules. They should e-mail or text only people they know. If they receive a mean message, they should show it to their parents or teachers immediately. This is a window of opportunity for parents. Nine- and 10-year-olds are still willing to go to their parents with their cyber problems. However, parents have only one opportunity to keep the door open. If parents respond without being judgmental, angry, or critical, then their kids might come back with further concerns. Ideally, parents can help kids compose responses or interventions to mean behavior they experience online. When possible, parents should encourage kids to be "upstanding" citizens and to respond to inappropriate messages by pointing out that the text or picture is mean and the sender should take it down or delete it. Explore with your kids why certain pictures and texts might make them feel uncomfortable. It may not be obvious to an 8- to 10-year-old.

Social Media for Kids

While Instagram, SnapChat and Ask.fm are increasingly popular with older elementary school kids and tweens, there are other social media sites that are child friendly. Child-friendly social networking platforms provide parental controls, restricted language, and are designed with younger children in mind. Other than Club Penguin, these sites are often fleeting, but here are a few examples of currently popular child-/tween-friendly sites:

- **Grom Social**: Social media site started by an 11-year-old. Kids can chat, share videos, and get homework help. Monitored 24/7 and parents receive report cards of their child's online activity.
- **YourSphere:** Kids can create Web pages and play games. Children can create groups called "spheres" to showcase their interests.
- **Kidzworld:** Social network for children ages 9–16. Kids can interact in moderated chat rooms and forums. They can create groups and write blogs but personal information can't be shared. Site monitored for bullying.
- **Club Penguin** and **iTwixie**, mentioned in Chapter 7 for younger kids, are wonderful for kids 8–10 years of age.

Can my 9-year-old have an Instagram account?

Technically, you must be 13 years of age to join Instagram, Facebook, and many (not all) social networking sites. This is because of the Children's Online Privacy Protection Act (COPPA). The law addresses how Web operators collect and use the personal information of children under 13 years of age. Despite the age policy, Instagram has become a popular entrée into social media. Instagram is a photo editing and sharing app that also allows you to post pictures to Twitter and Facebook. It was bought by Facebook in 2012 and has over 150 million users monthly. By default, settings are public but can be made private. Instagram is quickly taking over the teenage social network market and may eclipse Facebook among the younger set in this country.

Instagram Guidelines for Those Under 10 Years of Age

✓ Parents should set up the account; don't allow your kids to do it.

✓ Set privacy settings.

✓ Require children to ask permission to post pictures.

✓ Encourage your children to post about interests, and not just send selfies (self pictures).

✓ Don't allow personal information to be revealed.

✓ Follow your child on Instagram.

✓ Discuss with your child any inappropriate posts.

✓ Discuss copyright and credit with your child.

> If you allow Instagram in elementary school, use it as a learning exercise.

Instagram can provide a learning exercise on credit and copyright. When we were in school, we learned how to research and find the information. Now your child has endless encyclopedias to tap. Authenticity, plagiarism, credit, and copyright are huge pieces of understanding and using digital technology. Instagram can start the conversation about using others' artwork and pictures. Children between 8 and 10 years of age can begin to understand about taking credit for others' work and photos. Instagram provides an opportunity to start these discussions with your child. By middle school, your child should be having these discussions in school as well.

Here are questions to ask:

"Did you take this picture or create this image?"

"If not, who did?"

"Did you ask your friend's permission to post?"

"Did you give credit to the photographer in your Instagram post?"

"How would you feel if other people posted your artwork or pictures and passed them off as their own?"

Is my child ready for a flip phone or a smartphone?

Clearly we will discuss this topic with regard to every age group from this point on. Eventually, your child will have a phone, probably a smartphone. The question is when, not if. If you have a child with a medical condition or a child of divorce, then I strongly recommend getting a phone. Also, if your child is traveling alone and you have safety concerns, consider a phone. Often anxious parents will get phones at this stage. It makes the parents feel more secure. In Chapter 11, we talk more about anxious children and technology. Anxious children often use their phones as a security blanket against separation, strangers, or whatever situation makes them anxious. In my practice, I often help anxious kids to use their digital devices as tools to manage their fears. I ask them to be mindful of their growing dependency. In third and fourth grade, I would prefer that anxious children fine-tune their coping strategies before adding phones into the mix.

In general, wait as long as you can. In most communities, the phone floodgates open in middle school.

If You Choose to Buy a Phone for Your Child at This Age, Here Are Some Recommendations

✓ Do not activate the Internet.

✓ Put close friends and family in the contacts.

✓ Allow calls only to people in the contacts and monitor your child's call log.

✓ If your child is texting, monitor the texts.

✓ Remind your child to keep the phone in his or her backpack and not walk on the street holding a phone.

✓ Do not allow your child to use the phone during school. (As far as I know, there are no elementary schools that allow kids to use their phones during the day.) This becomes more and more tricky as your children progress in school.

Sexuality and Body Image: The Fantasy of Photoshop

My daughter is 9 and thinks she is fat. Are the Internet and social media making this worse?

As already stated, between 8 and 10 years, gender differences in technology use emerge. Specifically, boys will use technology for approximately 1 hour more per day than girls, all in video games. Boys play video games on phones, tablets, handheld devices, and consoles. Handheld device usage peaks around this age. Girls will play games less and less on handheld devices and consoles.

My biggest concern is not that boys are on their devices 1 hour more per day. My concern is the contribution of digital technology to distorted body image and expectations. While eating disorders are rare in elementary school, the seeds for body image distortion are planted. I am concerned that technology may worsen those images. In the next few chapters, I will talk about how to use selfies to encourage positive body image and how to understand and manage sexting. As children enter middle school and high school, their Facebook and Instagram profiles may define them. Pictures will be "photoshopped" into avatars of real men, women, boys, and girls.

Young girls enjoy the myriad apps and games that allow girls to explore dress-up and avatars. Avatars can allow the user to try out blue hair and yellow nails. I love games that encourage girls and boys to play dress-up. However, you should begin to point out unrealistic photos and images to your children. Today photos do not represent reality. They often bear no resemblance to reality. Kids need to understand how easily pictures can be manipulated and how that can lead to unrealistic expectations about body image.

A picture is worth a hundred words. Go on an online adventure with your children to show them how images can easily be distorted. There is a great story from the fall of 2013 that can illustrate this for your child. (You can find it at *thestir.cafemom.com* under their technology section.) A fifth-grade teacher took a picture of herself holding a note stating that her class was doing a study of Internet safety and asking if readers could "like" the image. The image went viral and users of Reddit starting changing the image and forwarding it. There is a pirate iteration and image where the teacher has been turned into a sleeping Morgan Freeman. More illustrative of the teacher's point, viewers were able to change the note to say all kinds of funny and inappropriate things. It is a great lesson about how posted images can easily be manipulated.[5]

My Recommendations about Fantasy and Photoshop

✓ Talk about "sexy" and "perfect" images with your children (boys and girls!).

✓ Ask if pictures of celebrities (both male and female) look real to them.

✓ If they don't look real, then how do you know?

✓ Help kids distinguish between "perfect" and "real."

✓ Ask if "real" can be beautiful. Find examples in your life.

✓ Show your children, firsthand, how photos or images can be changed. (Use the fifth-grade teacher lesson from above or take your own pictures and change them.)

✓ Focus on healthy body image in your home:

  ✓ Fit over thin
  ✓ Healthy over sexy
  ✓ Physically active over sedentary
  ✓ Real over perfect

The sex and sexuality stuff begins in third and fourth grade. The talk about gender roles and being thin and sexy is pervasive through late elementary school and into middle school. Most 9- and 10-year-olds are not overly interested in or focused on the opposite sex. However, there is teasing, crushes, and a growing awareness of intimacy and sex. Digital technology has brought "sex" to elementary school because it is so easy for pre-tweens to search for and find information on the Internet. Many kids will begin to learn about the mechanics and the realities of sex before middle school (especially kids with older siblings). Parents should try to stay ahead of the "birds and the bees" so they are not caught off guard.

The Birds and the Bees: "Sex" in Late Elementary School

Ten-year-old Rachel had a slumber party for her birthday. Her mom, Lynn, overheard the girls giggling and shrieking "Noooooo!" from the kitchen where she was getting ready to serve them pizza. When she called Rachel in to help carry plates and napkins out to the party, Rachel seemed subdued, and Lynn asked her if anything was wrong. Her daughter quickly said no in a way that told Lynn she wasn't going to say any more, so she dropped the subject but lingered in the kitchen. There she picked up enough words from the ongoing conversation to learn that the girls were listening to one of the guests describing what she saw when she caught her older sister having sex with her boyfriend. The next day Lynn bought a copy of a well-reviewed book about sexuality written for preteen girls and told Rachel that whenever she wanted to read it, her mom was there to answer any questions she had.

Not surprisingly, Rachel never said a word about the book, but several weeks later Lynn did her habitual check of their computer's browser history and found that Rachel had been searching "sex." The sites her daughter had found were a little more adult than the book Lynn had provided, but they were educational and even a little clinical. That didn't bother Lynn. What disturbed her was that her daughter hadn't come to her with questions. As a single mom, she valued the very close relationship she had with Rachel and felt sad and frustrated by being denied this important dialogue. So she made one more offer to answer any questions Rachel had and then let it go. Her daughter hadn't broken her technology rules. When she was curious about sex, she had simply gone looking for answers on her own.

Apparently, the "birds and the bees" discussion went out with Atari and landlines. The goal is to create an environment where there can be an ongoing dialogue. Access to information (and porn) has changed since kids sneaked into adult sections of the bookstores and peeked at their dad's *Playboy* magazines. Most kids begin this discussion in middle school, and we will return to this topic in the next chapter. However, if your child asks questions or has an interest, then the dialogue begins now. I am sure you are not surprised that Rachel went to the Internet instead of asking her mom questions. Kids go to the Internet for questions about their body and health. It is one of the greatest things about technology. However, you must help your 10-year-old understand that there is a lot of misinformation about sex on the Internet. I encourage parents to buy paper-bound books about sex and the body. I would tell younger kids not to search about sex unless with a parent. Having said that, the goal is to keep communication open. Lynn felt that reprimanding Rachel for looking up sex would result in shutting down the conversation. Of course if Rachel had landed on more inappropriate sites, then Lynn would have been forced to address the issue head on.

TAKE-HOME POINTS

✓ Your child's independent relationship with technology starts **now**.

✓ Your child is ready to internalize tech rules.

✓ Your child should play a role in developing a family tech plan.

✓ Your child has the moral development to understand digital citizenship.

✓ Parents' focus should be on defining and encouraging digital citizenship.

✓ Encourage your kids to bring you upsetting or mean texts and photos.

✓ Help your child identify "kind" versus "mean" behavior in the digital world.

✓ Child-friendly social networks may be a good introduction to social media.

✓ Your child will begin to communicate and socialize via digital technology.

✓ Children will learn about the Internet, social media, and games from peers.

✓ It is useless and misguided to completely restrict digital technology at this point.

✓ Children should ask permission to use devices and the Internet.

✓ Children must ask permission to buy, download, or join games and websites.

✓ Children need permission to post pictures or friend/follow people.

✓ You may give your child a phone, but he doesn't necessarily need one.

✓ Parents should encourage the use of digital media for education and creativity.

✓ Children should understand how images can be modified and distorted.

✓ Kids should learn to be wary about the authenticity of online information and images.

✓ Kids will learn about sex on the Internet (or through friends who learn about it on the Internet).

✓ Encourage your kids to come to you to discuss sex because there is so much misinformation online.

✓ The "birds and the bees" is an ongoing dialogue about sex, body image, and the Internet.

9 Tweens and the Texting Revolution

Digital Media Use at Its Peak

Ages 11–14

Brooke is 11 now, and we bought her an iPhone for her birthday in August. For a "tween" girl that was already obsessed with screens . . . she definitely hit the motherlode—and we have been floundering trying to figure out how to rein her in ever since.

We have tried to set some ground rules—of course they are very hard to police. Weekdays she is supposed to be off her phone from 4:00 to 7:00 P.M. This allows her a half hour after school to play around—and send 300 texts. It also gives her a little bit of time after homework, dinner, etc. She is supposed to be in bed at 9:00 with screens off so she can read and relax—and then lights out at 9:30.

This all sounds great, but the truth is her homework is often on the school blog, and she uses her laptop for her assignments. How can we know if she is responding to the endless flow of texts and e-mails or surfing the Internet when she is supposed to be focused?

Also, if she finishes her homework early, the first thing she wants to do is get on her phone earlier than 7:00 P.M. But this just encourages her to rush through her work. . . .

We have also noticed that she isn't interested in TV anymore. We long for the days when she couldn't wait to watch *American Idol*!

Now it's all about texting, Instagram, and countless mindless apps.

While I could sit here and complain forever about my daughter, she is a rule follower; so far she has respected the boundaries we've set up—of course with lots of kicking and screaming. But in the end she listens. I have her texts come to me on my phone, and what I have discovered is that she and her friends are junkies! She is actually not the worst offender—she has many friends that text all evening, often until 11:00 P.M. even on weeknights. On the weekends it's as if they have nothing to do but text. When Brooke isn't on her phone for an hour, she will often find she has 75 to 150 texts waiting for her! Of course they say nothing . . . and they are usually group texts.

I have good relationships with all of her friends' parents, and I know they have no idea what is going on. Of course, I don't feel comfortable ratting out their children—and Brooke would never forgive me.

The one thing I can say has been helpful about the phone is that it gives us major leverage! Whenever Brooke misbehaves, we have the perfect punishment—we take her phone away. Her behavior improves almost instantly. It's kind of pathetic, but it works!

On a positive note, she does often use technology in productive ways. For example, she is having trouble in her French class, so she came up with the idea to research French learning websites and apps. She found a number of helpful sites and started using them without even telling me. Also, she and her friends are collaborating on a "play" they have been writing together on Google Docs. I think that's pretty cool.

Sound familiar? If so, you probably are currently parenting a tween, a boy or girl between the ages of 11 and 14. This message came to me via e-mail, and of course I've changed details to protect the family's privacy, but honestly it could have come from any of the parents I know with a child this age. Digital technology use skyrockets and video game use peaks in the 11- to 14-year-old period. According to the Kaiser Foundation, total media use increases by **3 hours** a day in the 11–14 age group. If we include multitasking, there is an increase of **4 hours** of total media exposure from the elementary to the tween years. For these kids, this adds up to total media *use* of **8 hours and 40 minutes** and *exposure* of **12 hours**—half of the day!

OTHER HIGHLIGHTS OF DIGITAL TECHNOLOGY USE

- Cell phone ownership doubles from the 8–10 years, reaching 70%.
- Video game usage peaks in this age group at approximately 1½ hours per day.
- Boys are still spending more time on technology than girls, almost an hour more per day.
- Your children under 11 barely texted, but once they hit the tween years, they spend over **1 hour a day texting**.[1]

Although we're getting ahead of ourselves a little by looking at 15- to 18-year-olds (covered in the next chapter), if you take a look at the bar graphs below and on page 188, you'll see vividly that, with the exception of using technology to listen to music, 11–14 really is the peak of digital media use for kids.

LEAVING CHILDHOOD BEHIND: DEVELOPMENTAL MILESTONES FOR AGES 11–14

The goals for children ages 11–14 all focus on equipping your child to handle crossing the threshold into the far greater independence of the

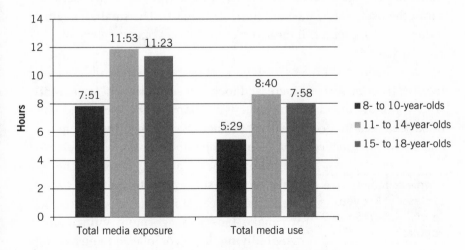

Media use by age. Adapted from Rideout et al.[2]

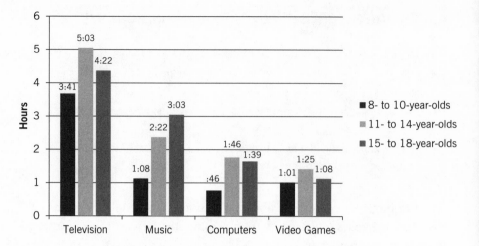

Time spent with each medium. Based on Rideout et al.[3]

teen years. Parents cringe when their kids turn 11. The cuteness factor for most parents is linear until their kids hit middle school. I like the term *tween* because it captures the idea that this age group is caught "between" childhood and teenage-hood. Your tween is less interested in you and more concerned about her peer group. She wants independence but needs you more than ever. Your tween may focus on his looks for the first time. He might care about what he wears or how much he weighs. Tweens' confidence fluctuates. They may feel great about themselves one day and horrible the next. The smallest slight or failure may trigger a full meltdown reminiscent of early elementary— but much less cute.

I probably don't have to tell you about the physical milestones for tweens, from puberty to increased focus on sexuality and appearance. And you may already be familiar with many of the social and emotional changes that come with this stage. Your tween may be moody and show less affection for you and for her other parent. With increased self-consciousness about physical changes comes a new sensitivity to rejection. At its worst, the increased need for peer acceptance can make kids this age more vulnerable to cyberbullying. It's a complicated journey, this

Middle schoolers love to classify: Are you sporty? Artsy? Smart? Popular?

jerky but relentless march toward independence. Digital technology can be a help and a hindrance at this stage of development.

Academically, school is getting much harder. Your child may receive real grades and assessments for the first time. He may experience the stress of middle school. His self-confidence may become linked to his academic performance. Your tween will have more ability for complex thought and a stronger sense of right and wrong. Your tween will be moodier but should also have the capacity to express her feelings in a more coherent and less "acting out" way. Some of the moodiness comes with middle school and the emergence of puberty, but occasionally it is a red flag for depression and anxiety.

With increased cognitive abilities and greater capacity for understanding, your tween should have a more sophisticated grasp of right and wrong and, along with it, a stronger ability to be a good digital citizen. While peer sensitivity can make some kids more vulnerable to cyberbullying, it's also at this age that kids develop an increased ability to identify cyberbullying and to stand up for others, to discern authenticity and be a critical digital consumer, and to understand the need to give credit to others for their work online.

> Eating disorders, distorted body image, and disordered eating all emerge for the first time in this age group.

WHAT DO YOUR TWEENS NEED FROM YOU?

At age 8–10, your child was just dipping his feet into independence, testing the waters. Now he may think he's ready to dive in—and may try to do so—but, as mentioned above, needs you as a life preserver more than ever. This is why establishing a consistent family tech plan that is also flexible enough to respond to your child's increasing maturity and independence is so important (discussed more fully in Chapter 12). Not surprisingly, as children spend more and more time away from the watchful eye of parents (and other adults), rules tend to relax. For ages 8–10 about half of families regulate how much time their kids can spend watching TV, and that number is reduced by half for ages 11–14 and then by half again for 15–18. Similar relaxing of rules governs what kids are allowed to watch. This makes a certain amount of sense. As children develop, they usually exercise better judgment about where to spend their time, and parents also become less concerned about their being exposed to inappropriate content. Tweens are capable of making good decisions about TV, but they still need their parents to provide scaffolding for other types of digital media.

Of course your ongoing role is not about rules alone. Helping your child develop a positive digital identity and become a good digital citizen is all part of nudging your child toward a healthy adolescence and adulthood overall.

What Your Tweens Need from You

✓ Help with time management online and offline.

✓ Protected study time.

✓ Protected sleep time.

✓ Coaching on how to use good judgment online.

✓ Help with sticky and uncomfortable situations online.

✓ Understanding of your family values about friendship, technology, and sex.

✓ Clear rules and boundaries online and offline.

✓ Parents who are good digital role models.

✓ Help with finding other healthy role models online and offline.

SCHOOL AND TIME MANAGEMENT

Digital technology will play a role in every aspect of your tween's development. The bigger question today is "How does technology not affect development?" By middle school, tweens will be using computers and tablets for schoolwork, and the distinction between academic and entertainment media will blur. A very organized mother of a fifth grader told me that she did not allow technology use during the week.

I have found that very organized, educated mothers often try for "no weekday technology." This authoritarian approach can work well until middle school. This mom received a handwritten (not e-mailed) note from her daughter's teacher explaining that her daughter needed her computer to finish her school assignments. So technology snuck back into the weekdays. Tweens will need to manage their time so they can manage school, technology, and the rest of their life.

Homework without Distraction

> **How should my tween manage technology and homework?**

We all found ways to procrastinate on our homework even without Instagram or YouTube. Today it might be even easier to get distracted, because a vibrating text is too hard to ignore when you are in the middle of the tedium of conjugating a verb or trying to decipher the periodic table. Therefore tweens must put away their phones when doing homework.

It also might be even more important than before for kids to do their homework in a public place, which allows for less distraction and makes it easier to get help when needed. I have found that kids are less likely to wander onto the Internet or fall asleep when reading and studying if they are out of their bedrooms. It is unrealistic to expect to monitor a preteen all the time or always use technology along with your child. However, the math problems are less likely to turn into Instagram if there is a chance that a grown-up will walk by and notice.

My Homework Recommendations

✓ Minimize distractions.

   ✓ Put the phone in another room.
   ✓ Have an adult hold the phone or tablet until homework is done.
   ✓ Have the child do homework in a public space.
   ✓ Keep computers in a public space (at least during homework).

✓ Minimize temptation.

   ✓ Start with homework that doesn't require a computer or the Internet.

   ✓ If that is not possible, start with homework that does not require the Internet (e.g., reading an e-book or doing math problems on a tablet).

   ✓ End with homework that requires the Internet (save most distracting homework until the end).

✓ Promote organization.

   ✓ Have your child go online and to a homework planner and confirm assignments before starting homework.

   ✓ Have the child (with your help as necessary) create a homework plan with estimated times for each subject before starting.

   ✓ Have your child (ideally along with you, at least at the earlier ages in this age group) look at a weekly or monthly calendar before starting nightly homework.

Technology as a Tool for Organization and Efficiency

I work and live in Manhattan, where some schools have the dubious reputation of being pressure cookers and Ivy League breeding grounds. I am often asked to help kids prepare for the academic demands of high school. It has become obvious to me that the kids who rise to the top of their classes don't always have the highest IQs or the most tutors. Generally, they are the most organized and efficient workers. Very few of us use Latin, Shakespeare, or advanced math in our adult lives, but we all utilize organization and time management skills daily. This involves both avoiding certain distractions and managing those we can't avoid. Tweens need to learn how to do both and to use technology efficiently in school and out.

Schools are currently in a transitional stage in figuring out how to best use technology for homework. Some teachers post online, and others do not. Some schools have homework websites for parents, and others have sites accessible only to students. There is also variability on when things are posted and whether homework should be e-mailed or physically handed in. Some schools have organized technology departments and curricula, and others do not yet have them. Schools are struggling to help students use technology to increase efficiency. I suspect that schools will sort out these glitches with time, but right now kids need help integrating school's online and offline expectations.

Can screens help with efficiency?

Efficiency and long-term planning are the cornerstones of academic success. Technology can assist us with both. As noted in the list of recommendations on pages 191–192, I encourage tweens to go online after school to confirm the assignments and then make a homework plan, writing out the assignments for the night and the time homework should take for each subject. I give tweens the option of starting with the easier or harder subjects as long as they get started, and you'll probably have a good idea of which will work better for your own child.

In middle school, I ask kids to work with timers so they get a real sense of how long their work takes and when they get stuck and why. My Homework is an app that creates an online school binder. Each class is color-coded and has short-term and long-term assignments. It can be linked directly to teachers if they have an account. Priority Matrix is an app that divides assignments into four quadrants, such as long-term/difficult, long-term/easy, and short-term/difficult and short-term/easy. It is a bit complicated for middle school but is an example of how technology can help students prioritize and plan.

I actually love Google calendar for middle schoolers. I encourage seventh and eighth graders to put their social plans in the calendar along with assignments. Parents can add events and view calendars easily. I like big-picture visuals and often advocate for poster-style paper calendars, but 13- and 14-year-olds are generally more comfortable with navigating screens than I am. I get more cooperation when I suggest that a smartphone would allow them to carry their calendars with them.

> David is a 12-year-old sixth grader who makes good grades and has lots of friends. He is a bit of a perfectionist and likes to be in control of school and his life. He used to get very anxious and overwhelmed when he had a lot of homework. His parents would sit with him, but he got upset and it took a long time for him to get his work done. Often, he didn't sleep well after worrying and procrastinating all evening about homework. In sixth grade, he found a creative way to use

technology to help with his homework. He found a classmate to be his virtual homework partner. He video chats with a friend during homework. He mutes the sound most of the time, but he can see his friend and ask a question if he needs to. He takes his friend with him via the laptop when he goes to the kitchen for a snack or to his bedroom for a break. They take 5-minute breaks and chat about school and sports. David and his friend are both determined students who want to be prepared for school. They keep each other on task.

OK, so study buddies are not a new invention. However, it is often not realistic or efficient to study with a friend in middle school. David feels less anxious and less alone. Homework is more fun, and he can get real-time support from his friend. At first his parents worried that it was too much screen time and distracting. However, David complains and procrastinates less if he can do homework on video chat. He is sleeping better and finishing his homework earlier. Technology has served to make him feel more supported and efficient.

IDENTITY AND INDEPENDENCE

Tweens are developing an identity influenced heavily by their peers and pop culture. Earlier in the book, I asked you to examine your relationship with technology. Now it is time to ask your children to do the same. Common Sense Media has developed a creative lesson plan entitled Digital Life 101 to help tweens reflect on their media lives.[4] They encourage teachers to create a concept map with four headings: Types (of media), Actions (ways to use digital media), Your Feelings (about media), and Your Parent's Feelings. Tweens are asked to identify the connections in their media life. After they complete a concept map, they are asked to create similes or songs that begin "My digital life is like a . . ." Digital Life 101 is meant to be a teacher lesson plan, but I encourage you to do this exercise with your children. It provides an opportunity for you to discuss your feelings and experiences with digital media. We want your kids to internalize your values and priorities along with the values they will be picking up from Lady Gaga, *Duck Dynasty*, and the "popular" girl at school.

After your tween has examined the components of her digital life, it is time for her to take stock. Pull out the logs that you used earlier in this book and ask your child to keep a log of how much time she spends on each component of her digital life—watching TV, texting, surfing, streaming, and playing. She might be shocked herself and choose to be more aware of her choices. As a parent, you are trying to foster independence by policing less and encouraging your tween to make good choices on her own.

> By the tween years, you want your child to internalize your rules and values and make good choices about digital technology on his own.

Is my child ready for a phone?

This is the first age group for which I would answer generally "yes." Middle school symbolizes the beginning of adolescence. Independence and expectations both increase. Kids often travel to school alone and spend more time with friends, with less parental supervision. **It is the smartphones and the subsequent texting that herald the beginning of your child's independent relationship with technology.** Cell phone ownership more than doubles from the previous age stage, to over 70% by middle school, and texting abounds. It is likely that your child will get a phone, and perhaps a smartphone, before leaving middle school. Having said that, there is no rush. Every child and family is different. If your child doesn't need one and isn't asking, then I wouldn't rush out and buy one. Be aware, however, that your child's social life may become linked to the phone. The phone is a mixed blessing and is the subject of much of the rest of this chapter. Peer relationships are an incredibly important part of this stage, and the phone will soon be in the mix of your child's social life.

If Your Child Has a Smartphone, Here Are Some Guidelines for Use

✓ Put close friends and family in the contacts.

✓ Parents must know *all* passwords.

✓ Start with having texts come to your devices.

✓ We love having tweens use Apple's iCloud, since everything comes to your device.

✓ Remind your tween that a smartphone is an expensive and valuable device.

✓ Tell your tween to answer the phone if it says "Mom" or "Dad."

✓ Make sure your child carries the smartphone in a backpack or purse.

✓ Don't allow your tween to walk on the street while talking or texting.

✓ Do not allow phone use during school.

✓ Hold the phone for your child during homework.

✓ Hold the phone when your tween is sleeping.

✓ Encourage your tween to actually speak in person to anyone she texts.

✓ Encourage your tween to selfie in moderation (more to come in the next chapter).

My last guideline I found on Janell Burley Hofmann's blog. It is the last of her 18 rules on buying her 13-year-old son, Gregory, an iPhone for Christmas: "You will mess up. I will take away your phone. We will sit down and talk about it. We will start over again. You & I, we are always learning. I am on your team. We are in this together."[5]

Let's Talk about Texting

> I've seen middle school kids spend all day gaming, texting, posting photos of their shoes to Instagram and then commenting online how cool they are—all the while sitting three feet from each other. At some level, it's harmless fun—just the new toy that this generation plays with. Except for when it's not.[6]

Texting has transformed the way kids communicate. Kids are more connected and less connected at the same time. The early printing presses of the Gutenberg era simply transcribed the oral tradition that was dominant in 1450. The oral tradition did not have formal punctuation; so many early books had run-on sentences with no commas and periods. Over time, the oral tradition transitioned into the written tradition.[7] Today we see a reverse transformation as we text and tweet. We use acronyms, memes, and pictures. Our communication style has increasingly become less wordy and more visual. It took hundreds of years to move from the letter to the e-mail and only one decade to move from the e-mail to the text and tweet.

Texting is the primary way that your tweens will communicate with their friends. Interestingly, when asked, kids say they do prefer face-to-face contact but find texting more convenient. Recently I commented to a parent that his daughter had not returned my texts to schedule an appointment. He asked if I had called her. I was tongue-tied (which is rare for me) and said that I had not thought to call her. At that moment, I realized that I no longer call my tween and young teen patients. I text them to confirm and reschedule appointments. Generally, they respond reliably to my texts but never to my phone messages. I realize that most kids don't check their voicemail, and if they check their messages they respond with texts. Kids often text each other to make plans to talk on the phone. Some kids have replaced the traditional phone call with video chat, Skype, or FaceTime. The phone call has become a more intimate form of communication. Texting and posting are more convenient and suffice for most communication needs. The intimacy of the phone call is reserved for the BFF and maybe the boyfriend.

So what's wrong with this picture? It depends.

How much texting is too much?

Some kids get so involved in texting and so distracted from everything else by incoming texts, especially group texts, that they can't seem to concentrate on more important things, whether it's homework or listening to their parents! There's no doubt that texting has, well, gone viral:

- The average teen (13–17) sends 3,339 texts per month.[8]
- Girls 13–17 send 4,050 texts per month.[9]
- Some kids send as many as 10,000 texts per day.[10]

A phenomenon known as **hypertexting** has been found to be associated with high-risk behavior. This is of concern considering that hypertexting is defined as more than 120 texts a day—it means 3,600 texts a month for a 30-day month, which means the *average* teenage girl is hypertexting. A study of 4,000 high school students in Denver found that kids who hypertexted and spent 3 hours or more on social media sites were at greater risk for smoking, risky sex, depression, eating disorders, drug and alcohol abuse, and absenteeism. The lead researcher explained that it makes sense that these technologies made kids fall into the trap of trying to fit in. If they are trying so hard to fit in online, then they are likely also trying to fit in by drinking or having too much sex. The Denver study refers to high school students, but the hypertexting and excessive social media use start in late middle school.[11] It can be hard for parents to figure out how many texts are "too many." Parents should use the impairment model. If texting is interfering with functioning or has become overly obsessive and leads to distress and irritability, then you have your answer.

Driving and Texting: Are Mom and Dad Texting While Driving?

Then there's the distraction factor: Tweens are not yet licensed to drive, although by age 14 many of them can't wait to get their learner's permit. Now is the time to make the case that phone use while driving, and certainly texting, is forbidden. A full 48% of teens have reported that they've been in the car with a parent who is texting while driving. This is the worst kind of modeling, and now—before your tween is old enough to drive—is the time to model putting the phone away while driving. The stories and statistics about the risk of car accidents while texting are legion; see the next chapter.

> **Should I monitor my child's texts and other digital activity? It seems like an invasion of privacy.**

I recently sat with a lovely older couple who each had a 30-year-old son from a first marriage. They expressed concern about the screen time of the 12-year-old boy they had had together. He was much more sullen and secretive since they had gotten him an iPhone for his birthday. I asked if they were reading his texts. They looked at me aghast! The mother said that she had raised a son and always prided herself on respecting his privacy. She had not read her older son's diary or listened to his conversations. Of course, he was 30 years old and did not have smartphones, texting, or Facebook until he was a young adult. I explained that the concept of privacy had changed in the last 15–20 years. Certainly the NSA and Google could read their sons' texts. College admissions offices have access to Facebook. It is an accepted fact that employers often Google prospective employees before hiring them. It is safe to assume that many people will have access to your child's digital footprint by the time your child is an adult.

> No one but a nosy family member or housekeeper had the key to the locked diaries of the 20th century. Today, almost anyone can have the key to someone's digital footprint.

Reading the texts of a 12-year-old is not an invasion of privacy; it's protective and educational. When you read your tween's texts:

- ■ You can view how he portrays himself and whether he is kind or bullying.
- ■ You can intervene and help him respond to mean texts even if they are not directed at him.
- ■ You can help him manage the onslaught of texts, which can become a huge responsibility.
- ■ You can point out when someone is being sexually inappropriate.
- ■ You can be sure that he deletes and does not forward inappropriate pictures that he receives.
- ■ You can point out how he presents himself online and make sure it is in line with his ideal self.

Some Recommendations for Monitoring Your Tween's Digital Life

✓ Have texts come to your devices when your tween begins texting.

✓ As your child gets older, you can monitor texts periodically.

✓ Friend your child on Facebook and follow on Instagram.

✓ Don't forget to check the child's social media sites regularly.

✓ Don't comment on your child's social media posts unless given permission.

✓ If you see less activity than usual, suspect that it's a phony account.

✓ Keep all of your child's passwords.

✓ Require permission to join any new social media networks.

✓ Require permission to buy any new apps and games.

✓ Tweens should follow the rating systems of games.

✓ Look at the browser history on the computers accessed by your tween.

✓ Look at apps and correspondence on phones and tablets.

The truth is that most kids can outwit their parents in the digital sphere. I work with one particularly clever 11-year-old boy who hacks his tablet and Android so his parents can't delete undesirable games and apps. Technology writer Ann Brenoff wrote about how helpless she felt when her middle school son contacted a stranger online. She works as a "technology expert" but couldn't protect her son. She lamented that she has resorted to spying. She "fights apps with apps." Kids use *sendvapor.com* to make texts disappear and Snapchat to make pictures disappear. They also use Wickr, whose tagline is "leave no trace."

Parents can counter with apps such as:

- **Txtwatcher.com:** Works on Android devices. It has mapping features to alert you when your child is texting. It flags cyber-bullying, sexting, and drug and alcohol language. It can also determine whether your child is texting and driving.
- **Mobile Spy:** Allows for broad monitoring, including text messages, calls, GPS location, website visitation, and photos taken.

I do not recommend these types of monitoring programs unless you already suspect mischief. If you have reason to believe that your youngster is hiding things from you, then you may need to resort to shadowing or spying. Middle schoolers need measured independence. Don't make the mistake of thinking that you can or must turn your pre-teens free. It is not yet time to set them free. But as a parent you have an opportunity to mentor and apprentice them before you set them free.

The goal is collaboration, not dictatorship.

SOCIAL PRESSURE AND CYBERBULLYING

Megan Meier was a normal 13-year-old who developed an online friendship with a boy named "Josh." After she had come to trust Josh, Josh began to tell her that no one at school liked her. Other classmates got involved in a name-calling exchange. She reached out to her mom, who was both supportive and frustrated. After a heated exchange with her mother, she went up to her room and hung herself.[12] It turned out that "Josh" was the 47-year-old mother of a friend. The mother was angry that Megan had been saying mean things about her daughter.

In September 2013, 12-year-old Rebecca Sedwick jumped to her death from a concrete plant due to cyberbullying. Guadalupe Shaw, a 14-year-old girl, was one of her tormentors. She had posted that Rebecca should "eat bleach and die." After the suicide she posted, "Yes IK I bullied REBECCA & she killed herself but IDGAF" (IDGAF: I don't give a F).

Cyberbullying is the use of electronic communication to bully a person. Usually, messages are threatening or intimidating. Cyberbullying includes mean texts, e-mails, or posts on social networking sites. Bullies can post embarrassing pictures and videos. Bullies can make fake profiles and pretend to be trusted friends. Bullies can also lure kids into trusting them and then organize horrible pranks or become abusive.

Here are some alarming statistics about bullying and cyberbullying:

- Approximately 25–40% of teenagers have been victims of cyberbullying. Preliminary research shows this number to be increasing.[13]
- Approximately 15% of teens report bullying others online.[14]
- 5% of high school students miss school daily due to safety concerns.[15]
- 70% of teens report that they have seen bullying online.
- 90% of kids who have seen social media bullying have not done anything about it.

- Only 1 in 10 kids tell their parents about being bullied.
- Girls are twice as likely to be bullied online as boys.
- Bullying is often a trigger for suicide attempts.[16]

Why is cyberbullying any different from schoolyard teasing and taunting?

You don't need to be a psychiatrist to know that bullying can be devastating and traumatic. Cyberbullying can be more severe than school bullying because you can't escape it. Children can often find relief from school bullying by going home. They often resist going to school to avoid the abuse. Cyberbullies can haunt your child 24 hours per day, 7 days per week. Texts and posts can also be distributed quickly and anonymously. The anonymity can create a false sense of trust as in Megan Meier's situation. Cyberbullies can reach a broad audience and are not always easy to trace.

It is hard to know who exactly becomes a cyberbully. Some kids cyberbully because they are frustrated, angry, bored, or curious. Others cyberbully to consolidate their social standing. It can be hard to do damage control with cyberbullying. You can delete mean posts or pictures on the device of origin, but once they have been distributed you can't easily delete them. Despite all of our talk about open communication and dialogue, kids often don't come to their parents. They worry about disappointing their parents. Parents are often critical of their tween's online behavior in the first place; therefore kids fear parental retribution if they go to their parents for help.

Cyberbullying can be more subtle, but still very hurtful.

Rachel is an 11-year-old fifth-grade girl who was bullied in school. The school and I were worried that she was being cyberbullied as well. At school, she felt there were three bullies and many followers. Some of the followers were her previous friends. She assumed they were too fearful to stand up to the "mean girls." By the current definitions of cyberbullying, she really wasn't being bullied. But no one in her class responded to her attempts to reach out online. She missed a good deal of school due to the bullying. She would e-mail longtime classmates to get assignments, and no one would respond. Presumably, she had been identified as the "victim" in the class, and the other kids kept their distance out of fear of being identified with her. With time and tears, she learned to manage the traditional bullying, but she was hurt by each unreturned e-mail or text.

Parents should try to identify cyberbullying because it can have serious consequences. It has been linked to anxiety, depression, low grades, poor self-confidence, and, occasionally, suicide.

Of course, there are warning signs. However, the media often exaggerates how easy and obvious it should have been to pick up on these "red flags." I want to warn you that these symptoms are generally broad and often nonspecific. However, parents, families, and friends should always be on the lookout for symptoms such as:

■ Declining grades in school
■ Social isolation and withdrawal
■ Mood changes
■ Physical complaints
■ Nightmares
■ School avoidance

These warning signs are very broad and hardly exclusive to cyberbullying. If you observe a change in your child's behavior, you should investigate. I would suspect cyberbullying if you saw an abrupt change in your child's relationship with technology. I would find it concerning if your child was more anxious or irritable when online. I would worry if she shut off the screen when you walked into the room or was more jumpy when online. This might be a red flag to explore with your tween how she is feeling about her digital life. If you have concerns, check out the tween's texts and social media sites.

You should take action when you observe any change in your child's functioning. Remember to keep bullying and cyberbullying on the radar. I ask every tween and teen who walks into my office about mistreatment at school and online. I don't use the word *bully* because it often connotes something more severe in their mind. I try to develop a digital foundation with each patient. I ask:

> "Has anyone been mean to you at school?"
>
> "Has anyone been mean to you online?"
>
> "Is there a lot of social drama on school or online?"
>
> "How do you generally communicate with your friends? Video chat? Text? Facebook message? Tweet?"
>
> "Are you a part of a tight social group or clique?"
>
> "Is the clique stressful or demanding in any way?"
>
> "Is there anything you would like to change about your current social life?"

I am a clinician, and these are basic questions that I ask most tweens. Parents need to tread a little bit more lightly or they risk being accused of nagging. Inquire consistently about your tween's social life. Ask for details and try to piece together as much as you can.

Cyberexclusion: Do You Really Need to Know That You Weren't Invited?

Cyberbullying is a big problem, but I see **cyberexclusion** as a more insidious daily occurrence. The public nature of social interactions has provided a new platform for jealousy and exclusion. When you were 12 and you weren't invited to the slumber party or the basketball game, it was upsetting. It was disappointing. Sometimes you didn't even know about the party or game. Other times, you found out months later. Today your daughter will see pictures of the party on Instagram and get a play-by-play on Twitter. She will know that her friends have gathered somewhere and she was accidentally or purposely excluded.

A 14-year-old girl told me that she was with her parents at a restaurant on a Saturday night. She checked her Instagram to find that her friends had gathered to hang out. She had not been invited. They were posting picture after picture. She sat at the restaurant glued to her phone, watching each picture pop up. She became very anxious and irritable. Impulsively, she deleted her Instagram account. She said that she would reactivate tomorrow but it was too hard to see every picture pop up. Some parents say to me, "That's life. My child needs to understand that she won't be invited to every party." While this is true, I am not sure that it has to be thrown in her face.

I have been struck by the myriad ways that kids can feel excluded. The 12-year-old who isn't tagged in an Instagram photo can feel hurt and excluded. The photo will have all the tagged names for all followers to view. All followers can see who is tagged and who is not in a photo. Adults often tag the people who are in the picture. But young tweens will post a picture of their new puppy and then tag their selected best friends. While it is OK to have best friends, this can feel like a very public exclusion to someone who wants to be or thinks she is close with the girl posting the picture.

Group Chats: Are You In or Out?

There are endless subtle ways that tweens feel hurt and isolated online (and in real life). I have found group chats to be a dangerous breeding ground for misrepresented and bullying behavior. Many tweens are not fully on social media, but they can join group chats. You cannot remove yourself from an existing group unless each participant physically deletes you. The positive side of group chats is that kids stay connected and can make plans. They can ask questions and get assignments very quickly. If you are on the group chat, then you are likely to be invited to any event that arises. The downside is the volume, content, and relative anonymity. When a parent reports that a child got 100 texts during a 2-hour screen-free homework period, most of the texts are group chats. Parents who read the chats will report that they are useless and lacking in content. Tweens will often get stressed by the number of texts that they need to respond to. Group chats have a mass mentality, so there is a real risk of your child being inadvertently pulled into mean behavior. The discussions devolve quickly. Kids impulsively post, and there is a large volume, so it is easy for someone to say something nasty and for many others to thoughtlessly and immediately agree or chime in.

What does online kindness look like?

Digital citizenship is about kindness. Digital technology offers parents a framework to teach their kids how to be brave and kind. Digital citizenship means being kind and brave. See the box below. Feel free to photocopy the dos and don'ts to present to your child as a reminder. Or try having an open discussion about them as a family, where you can brainstorm about how to respond if put in a position where it's hard to apply the dos or avoid the don'ts.

 The Dos and Don'ts of Digital Kindness

Do

- If you need/want to make a critical comment, then verbally say it in person, one on one.
- **Delete** mean or humiliating pictures/posts sent to you.
- Respond to texts/e-mails that ask for your help.
- Send kind texts.
- Stand up for friends who are being attacked.
- Unsubscribe from groups that are mean (if you can).
- When in doubt, do a digital reality check (see page 207).

Don't

- Post pictures of a party where some of your friends in the group are not invited.
- Post party invites/announcements on social media sites unless everyone is invited.
- Make critical comments about others online/on text.
- Take screenshots of Snapchats.
- Forward mean or humiliating pictures/posts sent to you.
- Hypertext.
- "Like" or forward embarrassing photos.
- Make critical comments about others online.
- Ask people to send you sexy/inappropriate pictures.
- Trust virtual friends whom you don't know in person.
- Pretend to be someone else online, even if you think it is a joke.

Digital Reality Check

Would you say or do this in the real world?

Could someone get hurt or feel excluded?

Would you want your grandmother to see what you posted?

IF NOT, DON'T POST IT!

LET'S TALK ABOUT SEX

I caught my son looking at a porn site. What should I do?

We started the sex and sexuality conversation in Chapter 8. The "birds and the bees" conversation looks different today. There is no awkward talk in your bedroom where your parents try to explain the mechanics of sex. The "birds and the bees" is an ongoing dialogue. Whatever you think that your kids know about sex and sexuality, they know more. This does not mean that you should get ahead of them and provide them with information that they are not ready for. Developmentally, kids are curious and other kids are talking about sex. However, kids (and adults) move through this process at different speeds. As I mentioned in the last chapter, if your child expresses interest, buy books and encourage the child to read the books offline to start. In theory, this allows for reading, questions, and verbal dialogue before they start Googling.

Whenever I start a child on medication, I have a "Google conversation" with the parents. I ask them not to Google because it will scare them and give them misinformation. I acknowledge that they may have already Googled or will not be able to resist doing so. In that case, I try to tell them what I expect they will find on Google—both the good and the bad. I ask them not to make any decisions based on their Google search but to come to me and I will try to address their concerns. As a physician, this has kept me very honest. In the past, a thoughtful physician might occasionally skip the mention of a rare or questionable side effect that could scare away a patient who desperately needs the medication. Not today! Honestly, I am not sure that this blind disclosure is always in the best interest of every patient, but it is the only way to practice now. This is the same with the middle school birds and the bees. You can omit whatever you choose, but they will see it on the Internet. It is much better for them to hear it from you before they find it in their travels through the Internet.

The conversation about sex and sexuality is starting younger—but that is not necessarily bad.

Tweens ask lots of questions online. They find out about menstruation, wet dreams, and homosexuality online. They often search to obtain a better understanding of their bodies and their sexuality.

The Third Google Click

It is the third Google click that becomes the problem. The first click takes you to the clinical mechanics of sex. The second click takes you a step deeper. Perhaps you will see nude photos or a video of a man and woman having sex. It is the third click where you get into trouble. I had a conversation with two parents who were deeply concerned about their daughter's "porn addiction." It was the third click that delivered their 13-year-old daughter to porn sites with pedophilia, violent sex, and images that truly dehumanized men and women. In middle school, kids are at very different stages when it comes to understanding and exploring their sexuality. Meet them where they are and get them talking.

How do you talk to your children about porn online?

✓ Don't punish them the first time you find them on an inappropriate website.

✓ Don't shame or humiliate them. You will permanently shut down the discussion.

✓ Encourage them to speak first. Try to understand what they know and understand about sex before starting any dialogue on porn.

✓ Encourage your tween to express an opinion about online sex and porn sites. You may not agree, but you will be building a dialogue and can provide valuable insight and education.

✓ Acknowledge how easy it is to get to these sites.

✓ Explain the difference between fantasy and reality. Porn is fantasy.

✓ Explain the difference between consensual sex and rape. Explain that some of the people on these websites are not willing participants.

✓ Explain the dangers of sex being linked to violence in porn and mainstream media.

✓ Talk about how porn can objectify women.

✓ If they visited gay websites, tell them about homosexuality and homophobia.

✓ Keep computers and devices in a public place if possible.

✓ Remind them that they are not old enough for "adult" websites and that you will be monitoring.

✓ Try to maintain an ongoing dialogue on sexuality.

Tweens have not fully developed their sexual identity and their sexual fantasies. While they may be embarrassed to come to their parents, they have lots of questions. Try not to personalize the discussion. Try not to tell them that they are not allowed to have sex with the same gender or that you don't approve of people who do X and Y. The goal of adolescence is to figure out what part of your parents' identity and values you want to internalize and what part you want to change. It is an evolving process. They need to know your thoughts and opinions. They also need to know that you are open to their views. Online sexuality and porn come up all the time. This is your opening to keep the dialogue going.

TAKE-HOME POINTS

✓ Total daily media use for this age group averages 8 hours, 40 minutes.

✓ Your child will likely get a phone, possibly a smartphone.

✓ Usage goes up and rules go down.

✓ Tweens develop their own relationship with technology.

✓ They need measured independence.

✓ They should understand parental opinions and values.

✓ Tweens need to be involved in decisions about rules.

✓ Tweens need to learn to optimize technology for efficiency.

✓ Tweens need to put away phones and unnecessary devices during homework.

✓ Tweens need to examine their own feelings and habits around technology.

✓ Tweens need help navigating sticky online situations.

✓ Tweens should talk about kind and productive texting.

✓ Parents should monitor their kids' texts, Internet, and social media use.

✓ Parents should confront their child if he or she is mean online.

✓ Parents need to try to keep a dialogue open on bullying and sex.

✓ Kids look at porn sites. They are accessible even with filters.

✓ Talk to your tween about the problems with online porn.

✓ Help your tween to take control of his or her digital identity.

Just Digital

**Rewriting the Rules on Independence,
Dating, Friends, and School**

Ages 15–18

Jake was 16 years old when he was referred to me due to concerns that he had "fallen apart" after his girlfriend, Zoe, had broken up with him. After the breakup, Jake had cried all night, isolated himself in his bedroom, and refused to go to school the next day.

When I met Jake in 2012, he was a stylishly dressed young-looking teenage boy with longish curly brown hair. He was friendly and didn't look depressed. However, he reported that he had been sleeping a lot and didn't feel like eating. He was a good student and wanted to be a writer/director and hoped to attend film school. He told me that he was in love with Zoe and couldn't see a future without her. They didn't attend the same school, but she was his main support for school stress. They spoke every day, and she knew everything about him. He got very anxious before exams, but if he saw her or spoke to her, his anxiety lessened. He explained that they were both busy, so they didn't spend as much time together as they would like. Occasionally he became jealous, but he trusted her.

I asked Jake about the breakup. He explained that they were having a minor argument over "stupid stuff" and she said she needed more space. She was feeling suffocated and felt that she needed to focus on school and getting into college. She said they should take a break. He panicked and started crying and found a bottle of his mother's pills. He put them under his bed but didn't use them. He didn't go to school the next day, and his parents became worried. However, later that night, Zoe had apologized and asked if they could get back together. Instantly, he was relieved and now felt that his parents were overreacting by forcing him to see me (4 days later).

I told Jake I was concerned that a breakup could trigger such strong feelings. I began to explore the relationship a bit further. I asked how they met, and he said "through mutual friends." I asked if they were having sex. He stopped, looked at me, and blushed. He said, "Well, kind of." I looked puzzled. He responded,

"Dr. Gold, we are very intimate and sexy. Technically, we haven't had sex in the physical way."

Again, I looked puzzled.

"We met online. We haven't actually met in person yet. But I am hoping that she can visit soon."

As a 40- or 50-year-old parent, you may be reading this case study and thinking that Jake is a troubled teenager. He is not. Jake lives in a New York City suburb, and Zoe lives in Sweden. They met through mutual friends and do talk and see each other daily. They Skype, video chat, text, and speak via Web-based phone. Jake is a B+/A− student. He is involved in theater and runs track. He has a group of school friends. He had a "real" girlfriend at the end of ninth grade who broke up with him. He felt hurt by the breakup and admitted to feeling safer in the virtual relationship that he had created with Zoe. Jake and Zoe's parents have spoken on the phone. Until the breakup, Jake's parents were supportive of the relationship. He was happy and doing well at school. He and Zoe lived in different time zones and encouraged each other to be social and "have a life."

Jake spoke to me for 30 minutes without any hint that it was all virtual. He did "see" Zoe through Skype and video chat. He did "speak" to her through text, Facebook, and Web-based phone. She was a strong support for him. He felt understood by her. They had what grown-ups would call "phone sex."

Jake is not the Goth recluse hiding in his room that you may imagine. He is neither angry nor alienated and gets along with his parents better than the average teenager. He does not have an "Internet addiction." Over time, he and I explored that he might be using his relationship with Zoe to avoid relationships with girls in person. He began to explore the anxiety he had felt when she broke up with him. Zoe and Jake "stayed together" until college. (Jake got a scholarship to a prestigious university.) Jake and his mom visited Zoe's family in Sweden. They are no longer "dating" but remain good friends and are in regular contact.

IDENTITY, INDEPENDENCE, AND RELATIONSHIPS: THE DEVELOPMENTAL GOALS OF LATER ADOLESCENCE

Your older teenager has increased capacity for relationships and intimacy. Teenage relationships are often intense and changing. Teenagers like to "try on" identities and explore different points of view. They have a more stable sexual identity and increased interest in sex.

Of course, independence is the end goal of adolescence, though sometimes teenagers who rush to independence get themselves into trouble. Unfortunately for us, teenagers begin to see their parents as real people with real flaws. They are brilliant at sending mixed messages to their parents. On a daily basis, I hear teenagers tell me they no longer need their parents. In the same breath, they will express anger that their mother can't find time for them.

Cognitively, their executive functioning skills are improving but not complete. They can set goals and develop work habits. Long-term planning is still a challenge. A very organized 17-year-old patient told me that her friends make fun of her for using her calendar on her iPhone. Planning ahead and tracking appointments is not "cool."

Teenagers are still prone to reckless behavior. They want to experiment with sex, drugs, and freedom. They don't always consider the consequences of their actions. Every season I have a teenager who actually sent the angry e-mail to the teacher that should have been deleted. Each week I see a teenager whose recklessness online gets her or him into trouble or causes some drama. Even though they seem more mature, kids this age forward the inappropriate picture, criticize friends on group chats, and spend too much time viewing party pictures from parties they were not invited to. Teenagers feel relief to have survived middle school. They report that the clique dramas subside after middle school. Teenagers feel a little bit more comfortable with themselves than they did in middle school.

> In my clinical opinion, the drama doesn't disappear by later adolescence, but it does evolve.

Along with independence, important developmental goals include the formation of a more established identity and more sophisticated cognitive skills. Here are some milestones your teen is likely to reach between the ages of 15 and 18.

- **Independence:** Your teen is definitely a man-child (or woman-child), showing obvious signs of increasing autonomy while at the same time still looking to you for advice and assistance:
  - ☐ Increased desire for independence
  - ☐ Realization that parents are not perfect
  - ☐ Possible identification with parents' faults
  - ☐ Shift from parents to peer group for emotional support
  - ☐ Desire to develop own value system and define oneself
- **Identity:** At this age you may be startled to see your teen becoming a fully formed separate human with
  - ☐ A greater sense of identity
  - ☐ An increased ability to explore inner experiences
  - ☐ An increased capacity for self-expression
  - ☐ A more well-developed sexual identity
  - ☐ An increased interest in sex
  - ☐ A greater capacity for intimacy
  - ☐ Frequently changing relationships
- **Cognitive:** The full set of executive functions in the brain continues to develop into the 20s, but by 15–18 your teen will have made significant strides in thinking:
  - ☐ More defined work habits
  - ☐ Greater ability for abstract thought
  - ☐ More developed executive functioning
  - ☐ Greater ability to set goals
  - ☐ Greater ability to think about one's role in life

TEENAGE DIGITAL TECHNOLOGY USE

Not surprisingly, as they become more adept with various digital media and have more freedom, teens' digital technology use generally goes up:

- 15- to 18-year-olds spend 8 hours per day with digital technology.
- 15- to 18-year-olds spend 11½ hours with digital technology if you include multitasking.
- 95% of teenagers are online.
- A third of teens report using an additional medium of technology while doing homework most of the time.
- 80% of teenagers online are using social networking sites.[1]

More teens report positive outcomes than negative outcomes from social networking sites.[2] Interestingly, they don't necessarily want to share what they are doing online—80% of teens say their social media profile is set to "private" some or most of the time. As you'll read throughout this chapter, not all parents feel they need to know about their older teens' online activity—only 40% of parents follow their kids on social network sites—and many relax their digital technology rules along with other restrictions as their teens approach college age.

Identity, independence, relationships, and schoolwork are critical components of adolescent development. In the rest of this chapter I'll review how parents can assist teens in using digital technology as a tool for self-expression, strengthened relationships, independence, and academic achievement.

DIGITAL FOOTPRINT: THE GENERATION GAP

If you were born before 1985, your digital footprint exists but may not be critically linked to your identity, relationships, or success in life. Kids growing up today will be somewhat defined by their digital footprint and it is likely to be somewhat permanent. While older people may not even care to create an online presence, teenagers cultivate their online and offline personas simultaneously and seamlessly. It is an essential skill that begins in adolescence and will evolve over their lifetimes.

How do I help my teenager with his digital footprint?

I am sure that your teenager is tired of hearing about his digital foot-print. His digital footprint should read like a portfolio, a résumé, or a calling card. It should exhibit your teenager's creativity and reflect her interests and opinions. I am amazed at the power of a positive digital footprint.

> Caitlin is a 23-year-old who sees me to help manage her anxieties about growing up. Recently she came in and told me that she was interviewing for a new job. She was asked to interview for an interna-tional startup company out of Asia. I was shocked, since most of my highly educated 20-something patients struggle to find even a medio-cre job. I didn't understand how this company had found Caitlin and why they chose to interview her, since she had limited experience (having graduated only 6 months ago). Apparently they had found her on LinkedIn. She explained that she had good Internet presence and knew how to network online. They came to her!!!

LinkedIn, the networking and job search social media site with over 230 million adult users, opened its doors to teenagers in August 2013 with the launch of the "University Pages." Teenagers can browse approximately 200 school profiles that showcase career-centric infor-mation such as a list of the school's notable alumni or data on where alumni are employed.[3] LinkedIn is an example of using digital technol-ogy to create a positive résumé. As teenagers get older, they are more likely to recognize that universities and future employers will care about their digital footprint.

Parents need to examine their teenager's online presence. They need to know what pops up when they Google their children. Armed with that information, parents should assist teenagers in creating and cultivating a multidimensional online portfolio or digital footprint.

How can my teenager use technology for kindness and social change?

It is important to have a good online academic and social résumé. It is even more important to use technology and the Internet for positive self-expression, for kindness, and for social change. HuffPost Teen blogger Patrick Mott posted, "Our social networks can tell a story about us and, if you're like me, you want to make sure that the story your Twitter or Facebook tells about you is a good story."[4] A few great examples include:

■ **Benjamin O'Keefe,** who started a campaign on *Change.org* against Abercrombie & Fitch after the CEO made a statement about targeting only "cool kids." He received 74,000 signatures and company executives met with him to discuss possible changes.

■ In May 2013, a Missouri high school student gained national attention for participating in Minddrive—a nonprofit group that inspires at-risk teens to learn about electric car design. They restored a 1967 Volkswagen and converted it to electric. They used a microcontroller device to program it to respond to social media input like #minddrive on Twitter and "likes" on Facebook. It became a social-media-driven car that was driven to Washington, D.C., to raise awareness about innovative education.[5]

■ **Zach Sobiech** posted a song entitled "Clouds" on YouTube to say good-bye to his friends and family since he was dying of cancer. The YouTube video was viewed by thousands of people and resulted in the formation of the Zach Sobiech Osteosarcoma Fund.

■ **Mary Streech** was in seventh grade when she was hospitalized for an eating disorder. Upon discharge, she started her own non-profit website to promote positive body image.

■ **Emma Stydahar,** a 17-year-old New Yorker, started a petition asking *Teen Vogue* to bring more real girls to their pages.

■ Others have joined **SPARK**, a coalition encouraging girls to speak up.[6] Since 2011, SPARK has taken action on sexual violence and unrealistic sexualized images of teens, including participating in the UN Tribunal on Girls' Issues.

> Teens don't need to make heroic efforts toward social change. They can simply "err on the side of kindness" online and in real life.

Teens don't need to change the world with their technology. They can help out a friend or raise awareness about an issue. The Internet has revolutionized activism throughout the world and challenged teenagers to be active and engaged digital citizens.

Digital Mirror: The Rise of the Selfie

> **My daughter is constantly taking pictures of herself. Is this a problem?**

A selfie is "a photograph that one has taken of oneself, typically one taken with a smartphone or webcam and uploaded to a social media site."[7] There was a 17,000 percent increase in the use of the word *selfie* in 2013. That's undoubtedly why it became the *Oxford English Dictionary*'s word of the year.

Teenagers take selfies all the time. They have become a way for teenagers to communicate without words, documenting a moment or an expression. Developmentally, adolescents are forming their identities and finding ways for self-expression. Selfies allow teenagers to have greater control over how they present themselves in cyberspace.

2013 word of the year: *selfie*

Still, parents and the media frequently complain that selfies and social media are harmful to teenagers. In my practice and my personal life I often hear parents express concern about the endless pictures: "My teenagers are missing the moments." "They are self-obsessed!" Ironically, selfies are actually popular among adults as well as teens, as you probably already know.

I agree that selfies (like everything else) need to be used in moderation. But keep in mind too that they may define this generation in a positive way. The selfie is a study in body image. Dove Soap produced a 7-minute video entitled *Selfie* for the 2014 Sundance Film Festival. I encourage you to watch it with your teenager (especially your daughters). The film shows a photographer going to a Massachusetts high school and teaching a group of girls and their mothers how to take selfies. The photographer says to the girls, "You have the power to change and redefine what beauty is. The power is in your hands because, now more than ever, it's right at your fingertips. We can take selfies."[8] In the film, teenage girls talk about how they take their selfies—worrying about how they come across, criticizing some of their features. The mothers learn about their daughters and themselves through the selfie exercise, ultimately embracing the idea that a selfie gives control back to the teenager and allows her to redefine and personalize beauty.

> **My daughter takes endless selfies but never sends or posts them. Is that unusual?**

I am not concerned about a teenager who takes selfies. I am more concerned when a teen refuses to take a selfie. This is similar to a teenager refusing to look in the mirror. Most teenagers take 5 or 10 selfies and accept one and post it without much thought. I worry about a teenager who ruminates over her selfies or refuses to take one in the first place. On the other hand, maybe your teenager is too cool for selfies—I can live with a teenager taking an oppositional stance for no apparent reason. Just be aware that refusal to take a selfie may be a red flag for body image distortion or eating disorders.

My Selfie Recommendations

✓ Remember that it's developmentally appropriate and trendy to take selfies.

✓ Encourage your teen not to selfie in excess but to use it in moderation.

✓ Remind your teen to embrace the moment, not the selfie—ask what was going on in the picture or why your teen had a certain expression.

✓ Talk to your kids about their selfies as a matter of routine.

✓ To learn about your teen's body image, ask how she picks a selfie.

✓ Help your teen identify how her selfies are unique.

✓ If your teen refuses to post her selfies, inquire about her ambivalence.

✓ Talk to your teenager about your own body image struggles.

✓ Model positive body image behavior for your teen.

IDENTITY AND SELF-EXPRESSION

> **I recently read my son's texts and he sounds like a gangster. What should I do?**

"Multiple personality" has taken on a new meaning in the digital age. Teenagers explain that kids speak one way online and another way in person. An Ivy League–bound 12th grader explained to me that he spoke the same way online as offline except with a lot more cursing. He showed me a few text exchanges. Yes, there were lots more swear words, but it was more than that. He did sound like a gangster. He used urban slang and made sexist comments. The text exchanges were incongruent with the well-dressed, thoughtful, and articulate young man sitting in front of me. I acknowledge that he may speak to me more formally than to his peers. But he acknowledged that he rarely used profanity and made derogatory remarks when speaking in person to his friends.

As an exercise, I often ask teenagers to look at their digital presence as a third-party observer: "If a stranger had access to your texts and messages, what would he think?" Most teenagers are smart enough to tell me that they neither cyberbully nor sext. However, they do not always think about how their digital presence reflects their true identity.

Ask your teen: "What would a stranger think of your texts and messages?"

Parents are often confused, hurt, and angry when they see their teenagers acting like "gangsters" or "hookers" online. The digital modality allows teenagers to explore different roles and personas. The anonymity and speed of technology leads to impulsive texts and posts and subsequently bad behavior online. Of course, your teenager must be mindful of privacy issues. But it goes further. He must be aware of the way he presents himself online. Parents have a great deal of trouble using restraint when they find their children behaving badly. It is a waiting game. As a parent, you need to be aware of your teen's digital identity and reflect it back to her so she can begin to see it for herself. If you can, try to withhold judgment and listen to your teenager. Identity development takes time and if you keep the door open long enough, she is likely to eventually walk through it.

Individual Self-Expression

> My son posted a picture of a serial killer, and his best friend made a positive comment about school shooters. Are they depressed or at risk?

The "links" and the "likes" that you share say something about you. Along with vampires and zombies, serial killers are quite prevalent on TV and in games. However, sharing links about real serial killers may not be such a good idea. There is a line between unpopular beliefs and violence and hate speech. Christopher is a bright 11th grader attending private school in Manhattan. Manhattan is notorious for being socially progressive and pro gun control. Christopher posted pictures of guns, explosives, and hate speech on Instagram. He was shy in school and didn't have a lot of friends. He wasn't bullied but didn't fit in either. Several of his classmates were concerned about his Instagram account and went to the school administration. The school came to me and asked if they should be worried about him.

Christopher's parents did not know about the Instagram account. They knew that he had a Facebook page with very little activity. When I met him, he was soft-spoken and very sweet. He told me that the school was being ridiculous. The Second Amendment protected people's right to bear arms. I agreed wholeheartedly but asked him why he needed to post pictures of explosives. He explained that if he lived in a different part of the country these posts would seem less inflammatory. He explained that the NRA had 3 million members and probably very few in Manhattan. He may have been right. His school had a very low tolerance for pictures of guns and explosives. They saw a quiet and isolated teenager with what appeared to be an online preoccupation with guns and violence. Although the school administration had made a lot of assumptions, it was hard to entirely blame the school for being overprotective.

While Christopher felt the school was overreacting, he did understand their concerns. Christopher and I examined why he was reluctant to participate in class and tended to keep to himself. It had nothing to do with the NRA. He deleted the pictures of tanks and the links to more extreme gun rights groups. Truthfully, he didn't care that much about the Second Amendment and the NRA, but his Instagram account made it look like he was passionate about both.

Christopher and I looked for healthier ways for him to connect to his community. He realized that he shared an interest in a popular role-playing game (RPG) and asked classmates if he could join in their game. He was passionate about politics, not violence. He started to post pictures and links about political issues that he cared about. They were more conservative than those of his peers but completely appropriate. His father encouraged him to make more connections offline, and his social media makeover resulted in a more authentic online identity.

Teenagers often enjoy taking unpopular stands and stirring debate. It is a normal part of adolescence to adopt opinions that are antithetical to your parents' views. Sometimes, teenagers need to hold extreme views before they can settle into a more moderate stance. I encourage teenagers to debate issues, but they must be mindful of their online presentation. Strong and provocative opinions can be misrepresented in the fast-paced world of Twitter and Instagram. I worked with a very bright Jewish high school student who posted inflammatory and anti-Semitic remarks and shared links to fundamentalist Muslim groups. Her school and her friends were concerned. She claimed that she was simply encouraging debate and trying to understand the opinions of groups who she felt were dismissed in her liberal Jewish community. I think she was trying to get the attention of her parents, who were distracted. It worked. The school and her parents paid attention. The school put her on probation, and her parents deleted her Facebook, Instagram, and Twitter accounts.

My Recommendations to Teens about Online Identity and Persona

√ Make sure your online identity matches your real identity.

√ Be thoughtful about what you post, link, and like.

√ Don't promote, endorse, or "like":

　　√ Hate speech (i.e., sexist, racist, homophobic)

　　√ Sites that teach you how to build explosives

　　√ Extremely violent sites

✓ Homicidal links or posts

✓ Terrorist or radical religious groups that aim to harm Westerners

✓ Anything related to wanting, buying, or selling drugs (including marijuana)

✓ Sexually explicit photos (naked photos of kids under age 18 can be defined as child pornography)

To be clear, I am not saying that teens can't have opinions related to any of the above. However, these topics are often misrepresented in a public space. Followers and "friends" may misunderstand or make inaccurate assumptions. Teens should be told to keep inflammatory discussions to real life or to themselves (and this goes for parents too).

Identity Development and Video Games

> My son is always playing video games in his room. Isn't he missing out on a time in his life that he won't be able to get back?

Stephanie and Jennifer are sisters. Stephanie is 21 years old and Jennifer is 19 years old and they attend different colleges. They are both avid gamers who tried to help me understand how gaming strengthened their self-esteem and enhanced their relationships. They have grown up with games and are both in healthy committed relationships with men they met online (as adults). When Stephanie was 17, the family moved across the country. She began playing World of Warcraft with her old high school friends. "It was better than talking and texting because we were participating in a shared activity," she explains.

Stephanie and Jennifer had grown up playing video games together. They started by competing with each other in racing games and expressed their sibling rivalry in fighting games. They even took turns, and each played the parts that the other was uncomfortable with in single-player games: Jennifer walked through morgues, and Stephanie swam in oceans. When Stephanie went off to college, they wanted to continue playing. They compromised and collaborated on games so they could have a shared experience. The games ranged from role-playing to capture-the-flag-type games and simple Facebook games.

Stephanie started playing World of Warcraft with "familiars" (friends), which is what she recommends for high school kids. As she gained more skill, she joined a guild of skilled players. She explained that there is downtime when playing and all the guild members chat with each other. They got to know each other, and eventually Stephanie met her boyfriend offline.

Jennifer plays more competitive games like League of Legends. She attended a convention for the game to watch and learn from those who play and commentate professionally. Conventions are moderated events with security and international players. Participants can meet each other offline and speak about their shared online interests. Jennifer met her boyfriend at a conference. Stephanie and Jennifer are excited about the growing popularity of competitive online games and e-sports.

Both women are good students and have meaningful offline relationships. They have active social lives and social networks but found most of their friends directly or indirectly through online connections. Stephanie and Jennifer are adamant that their online gaming experiences have strengthened their families, friendships, and relationships. They taught me how online games can be used for creative expression and social connection.

Multiplayer games can serve as a microcosm of real life. You can learn skills and independence. You can be a leader or a follower. You need strategy and alliances. You are rewarded for good work and punished for bad. There is increased recognition of the complex reasoning and skills needed to play these games.

> Young adults have begun to put their roles as leaders or moderators in multiplayer games on their résumés.

In competitive gaming, strong critique, verbal assault, trolling, and bullying take place. Stephanie and Jennifer feel passionately that their gaming experience has made them confident, quick-witted, and thick-skinned. They learned how to manage themselves in the games. They suggest that teens participating in these games:

- Use the ignore function (/block, /ignore).
- Report bad or disturbing behavior to moderators.
- Keep positive people around them (you are not required to play with everyone who asks you to).
- Take a break if they are no longer enjoying the game.

The generation gap is never clearer than when talking to teenagers and parents about online gaming. I receive a lot of phone calls
from parents who are genuinely concerned that their teenage sons are
"depressed," "doing drugs," or are "potential school shooters" because
they spend all of their time in their bedroom playing games. I follow
with a series of questions to the parents:

"What game does your son play?"

"What is his role in the game?"

"Is it a multiplayer game?"

"Does your son play with 'familiars' or strangers?"

"Is the gaming impairing his schoolwork? Extracurricular activities?"

"Does he have friends outside the gaming world?"

"Does he use technology in any other way (i.e., social media, coding)?"

I get silence on the other end of the line. The parents are concerned
about their teenager's irritability, stubbornness, and mental health, but
they don't really understand what their teenage sons are doing online.

Greg is a very smart 11th grader who plays lacrosse and runs cross
country at his private all-boys' school. His parents are convinced that
he is depressed. He plays games until 3:00 A.M. and hides out in his
room all the time. Upon meeting Greg, I saw a casually but carefully
dressed teen. Initially, he was soft-spoken and slightly sullen with poor
eye contact and had a seemingly arrogant demeanor. He brightened up
and seemed to relax when I asked him about gaming. I asked him if he
thought that his gaming was a problem. He said no.

I asked Greg to tell me about the game that he plays most. He
rolled his eyes because I am clearly not well versed in online gaming.
He explained that he is a raid leader on Final Fantasy (a multiplayer
game similar to World of Warcraft). He coordinates 40 people's schedules so they are available for the evening fight. He also updates them
on strategies and plans. It is a sophisticated game, and he enjoys listening to the input from his players for better strategies and the thrill of
victory with his teammates.

He explained that he generally plays with people he knows from school. Yes, he stays up too late playing. He does complete his schoolwork—he gets B's in school, though his parents would prefer A's—and has plenty of friends in real life, but he plays when he is bored or late at night. He said he was not depressed but was annoyed with his parents for nagging him all the time.

As a parent, you need to understand what games your teenager is playing. Sport games on a console are not too complicated to understand and manage. However, if your teenager is playing World of Warcraft or League of Legends, you need to learn more. I am not suggesting that you join the game (please don't), but you need to understand more about how he is using the game. Ask your teenager to explain the rules, etiquette, and roles. In World of Warcraft, your skill level is reflected in the details in your armor. In other games, skill level is illustrated by showing off a rare item or wearing a certain hat. Ask your teenager what he enjoys about this particular game. Is it competitive? Is it relaxing? Ask him to explain the violence. In some games women are raped and their heads are torn off in excruciating detail. In other games, players participate in medieval jousts and the defeated "disappear" rather than die.

Online games are a tool to express identity, create relationships, and work on independence. But of course teenagers should use games in moderation and recognize when gaming is interfering with their lives. Teenage gamers need their parents to understand how they use gaming. They need their parents to turn it off when they can't. They also need their parents to let them play when that is appropriate.

> Both teenagers and parents need to identify the merits of gaming wisely.

REAL FRIENDS IN THE DIGITAL AGE

Friendships in the digital era have an added layer of complexity. It has become clear to me that the "rich get richer" in teenage friendships that are heavily mediated by technology:

■ Teens who have social skills and healthy self-esteem are able to use social media and electronic communication to strengthen their relationships.

■ Kids with weaker self-esteem are more at risk of getting negative reinforcement. They may feel worse about themselves when they compare profiles and numbers of likes/followers, and seek reassurance online.

> **With all of her "friends" and "followers," I am concerned that my daughter doesn't understand real friendship. What should I do?**

Friendship formation is a key component of adolescent development. We know that face-to-face self-disclosure is critical to teenage friendship formation. We also know that friendship is highly correlated with self-confidence and well-being in the teen years. Texting and social media sites are not linked directly to loneliness, isolation, or poor self-esteem. Facebook friends and social media use have been linked positively to self-esteem. Social media sites and teenage friendships are a complicated marriage, however.

Selective self-presentation, self-disclosure, and investment seem to be the core components to understand about your teenager's friendships in the era of social media.

THE ESSENTIALS OF FRIENDSHIP FORMATION

- Social media sites facilitate increased self-disclosure.
- Restrained self-disclosure leads to strengthened friendships.
- Those who overshare are seeking reassurance.
- Those seeking reassurance may be more likely to get negative feedback.
- Teens with poor social skills are less likely to reap the benefits of social networking.
- Selective self-presentation can help teens cultivate their best sense of self.
- Overinvestment leads to disappointment and lower self-concept.

Selective Self-Presentation

> My daughter is always comparing her life to the fabulous parties and pictures that she sees online. Isn't this harmful?

The profile is the hallmark of most social media sites. It allows a teenager to present her best self. There is research to support the correlation between selective self-presentation and positive sense of self. So the ability to promote her best self in her profile could bring out the best in your teen. However, it is important for her to understand the difference between a Facebook profile and reality. You don't send your worst selfie or post pictures of the party you weren't invited to. "Facebook envy" is described as feeling sad or envious after viewing others' Facebook posts. Researchers have identified that the biggest triggers for adults are vacation pictures and birthday posts. There is no conclusive research for teens, but I suspect that not being invited to the party or the event is a big part of it. The goal is to help your teen to recognize that she can't be invited to all the parties but she can connect with friends, view profiles and posts with a critical eye, and feel good about herself.

How to Prevent Unhealthy Comparisons

✓ Point out the difference between a profile and reality.

✓ Help your teen recognize that she is seeing only part of the picture.

✓ Encourage the teen to focus on well-known friends—it's easier to idealize acquaintances.

✓ Show her how to focus on her own strengths when she begins to feel envious.

✓ Note that there is nothing wrong with adding friends and followers.

✓ Tell your teen that the Kardashians, Justin Bieber, and Beyoncé, who top the Instagram list, all have paid staffs who manage their Instagram presence.

✓ Remind your teen to turn off a social media site that makes her feel bad.

Self-Disclosure and Oversharing

The ease and anonymity of online communication make it easier to disclose personal information and thus leads to hyperdisclosure. This has been found to be truer for boys than girls. Self-disclosure is the glue that holds teenage relationships together. You want your teenager to disclose *some* personal information to a known friend when cultivating a relationship. The sticky part is that "oversharing" makes teenagers and adults vulnerable to disappointment, negative feedback, and depression.

For adults, oversharing is like what they used to say about pornography: "You know it when you see it." Most adults on Facebook have a "friend" who chronically overshares. She posts about her cramps, hemorrhoids, and depression. You know when she is having a bad day whether you want to or not. It is not so simple with teenagers.

Here are some questions your teens should ask themselves before they overshare:

> "Am I posting something appropriate for all my followers/friends to see?"
>
> "Would this communication be better in a single text or face to face?"
>
> "Will I be upset if no one comments or reassures me?"
>
> "Does my friend have time to hear my concerns?"
>
> "Will I feel better after sharing my concerns?"
>
> "Would I be better off venting to a friend or parent in person?"
>
> "Do I know the person well enough to disclose personal information?"

Investment in Social Media and Texting

It turns out that **it is not how much time teens spend on social media that matters. It is how they use it and their level of investment that gets them into trouble.** Research has found that teens with a high frequency of social media use are more likely to have a positive "self-concept." However, teens who are **overly invested** in their social media sites are at greater risk for low self-esteem and depression. Take two teens who use social media multiple times a day, one very invested and the other not. If social media is taken away, the overly invested teen may feel more disconnected and lost. The theory is that teens who become highly invested in their social networking site are less able to discern between the "social résumé" their friends present and the actual reality of these friends' day-to-day lives. Consequently, these teens use unrealistic and inflated comparisons when evaluating

Does Too Much Time on Social Media Sites Cause Depression?

The American Academy of Pediatrics (AAP) explains that Facebook depression "develops when preteens and teens spend a great deal of time on social media sites, such as Facebook, and subsequently exhibit classic symptoms of depression." Since American teens are losing interest in Facebook by the week, this should be redefined as "social media depression." In 2011, the AAP expressed concern that teenagers who spent a lot of time on social media sites were at increased risk for depression. Subsequent research has found that social media use is not directly correlated with clinical depression.[9] **It does not cause depression but can play a role in it.** In some circumstances, social media may contribute to low self-esteem and "unhappiness." Researchers at the University of Michigan followed 80 undergraduates on Facebook. They found that the more time students spent on Facebook, the less happy they were in the moment and the less satisfied they were with their life in general.[10]

Social media sites provide a new modality for envy, jealousy, and comparison. Social media profiles often present only the good and positive, not the real. Teenagers can quantify "friends," "followers," and "likes"—Facebook provides lots of ways for your teenager to ruminate. Rumination is defined as compulsively focusing attention on one's distress. The difference between rumination and worry is that the focus is primarily on the causes and consequences and not on the solutions. Ruminative behavior is correlated with depression and anxiety. Nevertheless, I don't believe social media *causes* depression, comparison, or envy. I think teenagers who are prone to feeling isolated and depressed may find that Facebook and other sites make it worse or become places for ruminative behavior.

themselves. This would explain why increased investment in social media puts your teen at greater risk for low self-esteem and depression.[11] (See the box on page 230 for more on social media and depression.)

To help your teens maintain a healthy relationship with social media, tell them that while comparison and envy are normal, profiles that look "too good to be true" likely *are* too good to be true.

Teens should be wary of judging themselves based on the number of "likes" they get or "friends" they have.

DATING AND INTIMATE RELATIONSHIPS

> My daughter is constantly texting her boyfriend. They never see each other or speak on the phone. Should I be worried?

Emma's parents scheduled a conference call with me because they were concerned that their gregarious 18-year-old daughter was in a bad relationship. They explained that Emma saw Luke, her boyfriend, only at school. They texted all day and night. Emma would worry if she didn't get an hourly text. Sometimes they video chatted before bed. No phone calls and no dates. Emma explained that they both had busy schedules and didn't really have time to hang out in person.

I explained to Emma's parents that their relationship was not unusual. Emma and Luke worked very hard at staying in constant communication but couldn't find time to enjoy each other in person. I reassured Emma's parents that Emma was healthy psychologically, yet I agreed that this style of "dating" was draining and not a lot of fun.

Dating doesn't really change, although the dynamics and the rules evolve a little bit with each generation. The current teenage generation claims to "date" less and "hook up" more. Texting, social media, and online dating have certainly revolutionized the way we meet and communicate around dating. There are also several types of dating:

- Person-to-person dating
- Formal online dating (e.g., OkCupid and match.com)
- Virtual relationships where partners don't meet
- Virtual dating with avatars (beyond the scope of this book)

Teenagers should not participate in formal online dating sites. Online dating has been a revolution for adults, but developmentally, even older teenagers are not prepared for online dating. It is critical to learn the social skills involved with dating and intimacy. Generally, I try to discourage teenagers from initiating romantic relationships online with people they don't know in real life. I think it is important to have experience with "real" people before starting to initiate intimate relationships online. If your teenager does get romantically involved with someone online, there must be parental involvement. **Don't shut it down.** Your teenager can easily hide it from you. Jake's parents spoke on the phone to Zoe's parents and spoke directly to Zoe via Skype. The emphasis should be on teenagers learning to navigate real relationships that will inevitably be mediated by text and social media.

I knew the times were changing when Ellen Fein and Sherrie Schneider came out with a new book in 2013 titled *Not Your Mother's Rules: The New Secrets for Dating*. In 1995, they had published *The Rules: Time-Tested Secrets for Capturing the Heart of Mr. Right*. It was a bestseller and generated lots of controversy. I was 25 years old, and my friends and I cringed at the idea. It encouraged girls to be "a girl like none other" and to play "hard to get." The feminist in me was nauseated, but I recognized that it is human nature to want what you can't have. "The rules" have greater meaning now since mystery and romance are hard to capture on Twitter.

Anticipation and longing have been the hallmark of romance throughout the ages. Digital technology has taken some of the "romance" out of relationships. One obvious advantage is that it is much easier to keep in touch if you are far away. My concern is that it is too easy to keep in touch. Texting, tweeting, posting, and Skyping with your romantic interest takes a lot of time and energy. It is easy to misread Snapchats. Adolescents are already uncomfortable with their sexuality, and digital technology adds another layer of uncertainty. Self-disclosure is easier, but that sometimes leads to sexting.

Every day, I work with a teenager or young adult who is obsessing about when to text back or whether to change his or her dating status. Last week, I met with Adam, who has been pursuing a new girl. He was frustrated because he really liked her but she sent mixed messages via text. She was always the last to text and never texted late at night.

Sometimes she waited 8 hours (she has a job) to return a text. He was getting frustrated and uncomfortable with the uncertainty. His friends told him she wasn't interested. However, she was eager to make plans and excited to see him. I asked him, "If texting didn't exist, would she be sending clearer messages and would you feel less anxious about pursuing her?" He looked at me like I was an idiot but gave me a resounding "yes." I have no idea whether this young woman is right for Adam, but she is not in constant contact with him. She is taking her time and creating excitement.

I routinely ask teenagers and young adults to imagine dating without texting and social media. Imagine having to pick up the phone to make plans. Imagine having to run home and listen to a family answering machine to see if your crush has called. Taylor Casti, an NYU graduate student, posted a funny spoof on the current state of dating. She wrote, " 'Wouldn't it be so much easier to arrange this [a date] with a five-minute phone call instead of a three-day texting conversation?' you ask. Of course it would. But it's 2013. These options just aren't available to you anymore."

It is texting and sexting that have changed the dating landscape for teenagers the most. Texting has completely replaced the phone when it comes to dating. When a teenager says, "he said, she said," you should always assume that she was texting unless told otherwise.

> "Said" has been redefined to encompass any form of real or virtual communication.

Your teenager does need assistance in managing the communication with a romantic interest.

Basic Guidelines for Teenage Romantic Texting

✓ Couples or "wannabe" couples should not be in constant contact.

✓ Texting should be used to make and clarify real plans.

✓ Real issues should be talked about in person (or at least with FaceTime).

✓ If a partner gets irritable or annoying on text, clarify what's going on in person.

✓ The couple's Internet presence and relationship should be discussed:

  ✓ Will you change your status?

  ✓ Will you post on each other's wall?

  ✓ How can texting exchanges end?

✓ Texting breaks need to be taken.

✓ If you have to get off, you can always blame it on your parents if necessary.

✓ If a relationship feels like too much work then take text breaks.

✓ Try not to text or post anything too personal.

✓ Don't text or post anything that you wouldn't want others to see.

✓ Resist "picture pressure."

✓ Don't Snapchat or text overly sexy or partially nude photos.

✓ High school couples break up, so don't send nude pictures!!

Sexting

> **My son told me that he received a partially nude picture from a girl who likes him. He wants to know what to do. What do I tell him?**

Your son received a "sext" from his admirer. Sexting is part of the fabric of adolescence today. Sexting is defined as sending sexually suggestive photos via text or Internet.

SEXTING STATS

- 10–20% of teens have sent or posted nude or seminude photos.
- 30% of 17-year-olds have received suggestive photos.
- 40% of girls who sexted meant it as a joke.
- 30% of boys who received sexts thought the girl expected to date or hook up in the future.
- Girls are slightly more likely to sext (18% of boys and 22% of girls in one study).[12]

- 30% of teenagers who sent a sext did so despite having knowledge of the legal implications.[13]
- There has been successful prosecution for child pornography for sending suggestive images of minors.

Teenagers who sext are not mentally ill or outcasts. They reflect a cross-section of all teenagers today. Sexting has not been linked to mental health disorders, but it has been correlated with impulsivity and substance use. Some studies show that boys and girls send sexts equally, and other studies show that girls are more likely to send or post a sext. Girls definitely feel more pressure to be "sexy" and more pressure to please friends and boyfriends by posting inappropriate pictures.

Developmentally, sexting is part of the process of identity formation and sexual experimentation. It is more dangerous for teenagers since they are more likely to be impulsive and less likely to think about consequences. Peer pressure to sext is high. *Thatsnotcool.com* provides teens with a creative, and somewhat silly, approach to online pressure. They refer to sexting as "pic pressure." They provide "callout cards" that teens are encouraged to share to help them defuse online pressures ranging from oversharing to sexting. The callout card for (or against, actually) sexting says "When you pressure me for nude pics, I throw up in my mouth a little."

Electronic Hickey

The pressure to be "sexy" is not new. It starts younger because there is more access to "sexiness." My 5-year-old daughter, Addison, chose "Gangnam Style" by Psi for her kindergarten playlist. It is the catchy dance song with Korean lyrics that sparked its own dance moves. The only discernible English words are "sexy ladies." She loves "sexy ladies" and walks around the house telling everyone that she is a "sexy lady." When I try to explain that she shouldn't be a "sexy lady," it becomes an exercise in obfuscation. I make circular arguments that little girls shouldn't be "sexy." I tell her that she should be defined by and valued for her brains. She gives me her devilish grin and puts her hands on her hips and begins the horse-gallop dance step that the song popularized. Sexy means dancing, rock star, and "fancy" to her.

By middle school, girls are often defined by their "sexiness." It is everywhere in pop culture. One study found that 50% of older teen girls who sexted did it as a "sexy present" for their boyfriends. Both boys and girls report pressure to sext, but the pressure is much stronger for teenage girls. In 2011 the *New York Times* reported on an eighth-grade girl who sent her boyfriend a naked picture. When they broke up, he forwarded it to another girl, who reposted it with the caption "Ho Alert, If you think this girl is a whore, then text it to all of your friends." It went viral in their school. The ex-boyfriend and ex-friend were handcuffed and spent the night in the county juvenile detention center. Three kids who had spread the picture were charged with dissemination of child pornography, which is a felony. One of the attorneys explained that having a naked picture of your significant other on your cell phone is an advertisement that you're sexually active to a degree that gives you status; it's an "electronic hickey."[14] Three years later, the same legal consequences are still being imposed: in January 2014 a 16-year-old girl was found guilty of child pornography for distributing nude photos of her boyfriend's ex-girlfriend.

> Kids in the United States caught spreading sexually suggestive photos have been brought up on charges of distribution and possession of child pornography.

Psychologically, sexting can be devastating and humiliating. Teenagers trust their friends and don't think about how easy it is to forward and comment on photos. Snapchat is one of the worst culprits. Photos are set to "disappear" after 0 to 10 seconds, but there is usually time for a screenshot.

> Warn your teens not to send any pictures that they would not want forwarded.

INDEPENDENCE

> I love that my daughter texts me all the time, but should I be worried about her independence?

Like everything, texting your mom constantly has its pros and cons. Hara Estroff Marano called the cell phone an "eternal umbilicus" in her article "Nation of Wimps." When you are growing up, you internalize an image of Mom and Dad and the values that they imparted through

No Sleeping with Phones

I said it in earlier chapters, and I'll say it again here: I feel it is important that teens never start sleeping with their phone. They need a break from parents, friends, schoolwork, and, most importantly, **the phone.** Try setting up a family charging station in the kitchen or den so that you can model this behavior as well.

the years. Then, whenever you find yourself facing uncertainty or difficulty, you call upon the "wise adults" that you have been privileged to know.[15] Teenagers don't need to internalize their parents. They can internalize "Text Mom and Dad."

I like the fact that teenagers and young adults can easily stay in touch with their parents. I love that parents can feel a sense of safety by keeping tabs on their kids via text. But parents often forget that the goal of adolescence is to foster independence. Teenager hypertexting can undermine the confidence needed for healthy independence.

My Recommendations on Parent–Teenager Texting

✓ Teenagers should text their parents when out at night.

✓ Teenagers should text their parents if they expect to be home later than planned or than their curfew.

✓ Teenagers should text their parents if they get into uncomfortable situations and need support (e.g., drunk driving, too much alcohol, uncomfortable party).

✓ Teenagers do not need to text their parents when they arrive at every location.

✓ Teenagers do not need to give their parents half-hour updates when they are separated.

✓ Teenagers need to turn off the car GPS and use a map once.

✓ In urban areas, teenagers need to take public transportation on their own.

✓ Teenagers need to be encouraged to set up and attend appointments on their own (when appropriate).

✓ Parents can respond to frequent texts but should encourage teenagers to make small decisions on their own (e.g., chai latte vs. skinny Frappuccino?).

✓ On occasion, teenagers should be safely separated from their parents without their phones (at a sleepover, on a Sunday afternoon outing).

✓ I love summer camp and programs that don't allow cell phones.

✓ **Don't overtext your teenager!!!!!**

TEENAGER RULES

Is my teenager too old for family technology rules?

Teenagers have fewer and fewer rules about the amount of time they spend watching TV and digital devices. They also have fewer restrictions on what they do and see online. I believe strongly in passing the torch and giving your teenager more freedoms. The digital world is more complicated for teenagers, however, and parents need to be involved and likely need more guidelines than are already in place. With younger kids, parents are more involved and kids are less savvy. High school is not the time to stop with the rules. Most parents start with the dating, alcohol, and curfew rules. A study for the Pew Internet and American Life Project found that teens rely heavily on their parents for advice about online behavior and coping with challenging experiences. Even if parents are setting fewer rules, they continue to talk to their teens about the nontechnical components of their online experiences. Sixty percent of teens report that their parents have checked their social network profile.[16] Checking and following your teen may lead to more immediate conflict but will ultimately result in a safer and healthier online experience for your teenager. I recently reassured a mother that it was not her fault that her daughter had started using cocaine and ketamine. She smiled at me and said, "Yes that may be true, but if I had picked up her phone just once, I would have seen the flurry of texts. *Just once.*"

ACADEMICS AND DIGITAL TECHNOLOGY

> How can my teenager manage the demands of school and the demands of technology?

There are four parts to the school discussion:

1. Schools in transition
2. How technology has changed learning
3. Time management and distraction
4. Sleep

Students in high school during the second decade of this century are part of an experiment. Technology is part of the core curriculum for the public schools, but it is being integrated in a slightly different way by every high school and teacher. Some students do all their math work on a tablet, others are not allowed tablets for math.

Ninth grade has always been a big transition year. Starting high school often means changing schools and having increased academic independence. Freshman orientation for parents and students should include an overview of how technology is used. Teenagers need to know:

- Is all homework posted on a single school server?
- What is the cutoff time for teachers to post homework and assessments?
- How should assignments be turned in?
- How can a student confirm that an e-mailed assignment has been received?
- Are laptops and tablets permitted or required in class?
- What are the policies on copyright and plagiarism?

At the moment, the territory isn't well charted. And if you can't figure it out, then your teenager can't either. Teenagers report that they've e-mailed papers to teachers who claim not to have received them. I often hear that teenagers didn't check the school website and therefore missed a late-posted assignment. There is basically a debate over every element of academics and technology. Is math work more easily done and understood on a tablet or a scrap of paper? Should all homework be posted on a single server? Should teenagers have Internet access during the school day? Over time, schools will develop consistent policies where all teachers take the same approach. For now, your teenager needs to understand each teacher's approach and have an integrated plan.

> ### How has technology changed learning and research in high school?

Obviously, the Internet has made research much more efficient and accessible. The question is no longer "Can I find the answer?" but "Which answer should I choose?" Authenticity and plagiarism are the key issues pertaining to research. By authenticity I mean the trustworthiness of the information posted on the site. Students need to assess where they find information and judge the value of the source. Being at the top of a Google list doesn't mean the information is superior to sites listed further down. In fact, many of those "first sites" use marketing and Google ad words to get to the top of the search results. There are also more and less trusted sites. The *New York Times* website and the National Institutes of Health websites are examples of well-vetted sites. Teenagers should be more wary of sites run by little-known sources, individuals, and marketers. Teenagers often trust websites too easily. Good questions to ask include whether the purpose of the site is sales or research and education. Teenagers should inquire about the credentials of the blogger and the author. Do they work for a marketing firm or are they writing their dissertation? In medicine, we use the peer-reviewed research model as the gold standard. Peer-reviewed research is read and assessed by experts in the field before being accepted for publication. It represents the best research practices. If there is peer-reviewed research to support a statement, then I am more likely to trust the information. Teenagers are very savvy technology consumers, but they are not always taught how to distinguish the trash from the treasures in cyberspace.

The Internet has made it possible for virtually anyone to reach the public, and the sheer volume of offerings online has made it difficult for all of us to separate the worthy from the unworthy. It has also blurred the line between what is original and what is not. People readily copy and paste material from websites into their own documents without regard for the copyright notice at the bottom of the web page. And the opposite happens as well, with websites and blogs pasting published material into their pages with abandon. The ease of access might make it tough for a teenager to keep in mind that schools expect original thinking and original writing. In 1985, plagiarism meant copying verbatim from the *World Book Encyclopedia* or buying a prewritten paper from someone at school. Plagiarism and copyright infringement are much easier to engage in and more prevalent now. It is important for teenagers to give credit to others and to take credit themselves for what they write and create online.

According to a 2010 study done by the Joseph Institute Center for Youth Ethics, **one in three** students has used the Internet to plagiarize.[17] There are now services that students, teachers, and writers can buy that review your work for copyright infringement and plagiarism. According to Turnitin, a paid plagiarism checker service, the top plagiarism sites are Wikipedia, Yahoo Answers, Answers.com, and eNotes. Helping kids understand the difference between paraphrasing, quoting, and summarizing is key to writing and research in the 21st century. I believe it is the school's responsibility to discuss plagiarism and copyright infringement. I also believe that teachers and schools should help students learn how to use Wikipedia and the cut-and-paste option wisely. Parents can proofread papers and stress the importance of turning in original work. The goal is to help your teenager take credit for her work and give appropriate acknowledgment to others' ideas and work.

> The most plagiarized sites include Wikipedia, Yahoo Answers, Answers.com, and eNotes.

Interruption Technologies

> **My daughter is always online checking Twitter and texts. How can I stop this from preventing her from completing her homework?**

Developmentally, it is time for your teenager to take control of her academics, including her homework. Because technology can be a distraction in addition to an aid, I think it's still wise for older teens to limit their digital technology use while concentrating on academic work. However, teenagers must gain insight and develop awareness of what is distracting and what is helpful to their academic success.

I Encourage Teenagers to . . .

✓ Voluntarily give up their phone during homework.

✓ Let friends know they are offline for 1 or 2 hours per school night while doing homework.

✓ Voluntarily do homework in a public space (to prevent distraction).

✓ Voluntarily use timers and make study plans.

✓ Use a big sheet of paper or digital calendar to plan out assignments for each month.

✓ Use the Priority Matrix app to help them prioritize assignments.

✓ Recognize when assignments and assessments are making them anxious.

✓ Recognize when they don't understand a subject and get help from a teacher, tutor, or friend several days before an exam or paper deadline.

✓ Understand that long-term planning and organization are infinitely more important life skills than calculus or Latin.

You have to cultivate a measured level of independence in your teens. Adolescents need to internalize a work ethic. It is easy to spot a teenager who is studying and working hard to please parents versus someone doing it for himself or herself. The goal for high school is to internalize the work ethic. Trust your kids and be willing to let them fail (a little bit) for them to grow.

Digital Dos and Don'ts for Teens

Do

- View your digital footprint as an online portfolio.
- Be kind when online.
- "Like" the posts and sites of friends you care about.
- Selfie in moderation.
- Communicate with your friends online.
- Create a rich and creative personal profile.
- Take breaks from texting and games when exhausted, upset, or frustrated.
- Discuss with your partner the "rules" around texting and social media.
- Text your parents regularly.
- Use technology to make plans and keep in touch.
- Set your own time limits for games and social media.
- Use technology for keeping organized and doing homework.
- Keep an offline or paper diary to document your deepest thoughts.
- Use technology for friendships, social plans, homework, writing, creativity, music, information, and social change.

Don't

- Forget that your digital footprint has consequences in the future.
- Say things online that you wouldn't say in person.
- Like or endorse sites that are racist, sexist, X-rated, or violent.
- Over-selfie.
- Overshare or sext.
- Believe that profiles accurately represent the reality of a person's life.
- End relationships on text or social media.
- Forward embarrassing pictures after you break up.
- Text your mother every time you need to make a small decision.
- Text and drive.
- Study with your phone and social media nearby.
- Sleep with your phone.
- Post your most sacred and secret thoughts.

TAKE-HOME POINTS

✓ You need to understand how your teenager is using digital technology.

✓ You need to continue to monitor the quantity and quality of his or her online activity. Don't give up on the rules now!

✓ Google your teen and help him to manage his footprint.

✓ Don't overtext your teen. Encourage her to make her own decisions.

✓ Ask your teen about her selfies, especially if she doesn't selfie.

✓ Point out the difference between reality and the selective presentation on social media. (Use friends' profiles as examples.)

✓ Ask your teen what a stranger would think of his posts, texts, and social media activity.

✓ Forget about your childhood diary; privacy doesn't exist in the same way.

✓ If you find that your teen is sexting, try not to get angry. Try to better understand his or her pressures, anxiety, and other high-risk behaviors.

✓ Intervene if your child begins to "like" or endorse hateful sites or comments online.

✓ Look for signs of social media depression.

✓ Don't be afraid to turn off the Internet, phones, games, or texting if your teen cannot.

✓ Set up a family nighttime charging station in a common room.

✓ Model a healthy relationship with technology.

ONE SIZE DOES NOT FIT ALL

The Digitally Challenging Child

Modifying the Rules for Kids with ADHD, Anxiety, and Depression

Dylan's mom and I cajole Dylan, a 7-year-old second grader, to come into my office. After reluctantly agreeing, he makes a beeline for my desk and computer. After spinning around on my desk chair a few times, he opens up Minecraft on my computer and shows me the new water slide that he has built. I have a hard time getting him off the computer. He is fidgety and walks over to my Playmobil toy hospital and trashes it in 20 seconds flat. Eventually, his mom and I convince him to sit on the sofa and his mom hands him his 3D DS. He starts playing and is lost to us. He is neither fidgety nor oppositional; he is transfixed by the screen. His mom begins to tell me that he becomes violent with his little sister after watching too much TV. He throws tantrums when she turns off games or the computer. During our discussion, Dylan looks up occasionally and is clearly listening to our exchange. When I tell him that it is time to leave, he doesn't budge. He doesn't want to leave.

In my office I observe that children and adolescents have different relationships with technology. Some children can play video games without parental conflict, and other children melt down every day when it is time to unplug. Some teenagers use social media to feel more connected, and others use it to hide from real-life interactions. Knowing your child's strengths and weaknesses is a key to being a good parent. Digital media has given us another lens through which to view our children and ourselves. The way your child uses digital technology may be a window into his mental health and general well-being.

> **The way your child uses digital technology may be a window into his mental health and general well-being.**

DIGITAL TECHNOLOGY AND ADHD SYMPTOMS

> Is every 7-year-old boy addicted to video games? Do all little boys become more revved up after playing games and watching TV?

Most children, who play games in moderation, don't become violent. "One size does not fit all" is true for digital technology. Children and teens who meet criteria for ADHD or who exhibit symptoms of ADHD are at greater risk of problematic technology use. As a child and adolescent psychiatrist, I am very focused on making accurate diagnoses of ADHD. However, for our purposes, the exact diagnosis is less important than whether your child's symptoms resemble the overall picture of the syndrome.

Does your child have problems paying attention?

- Does your child frequently forget to bring home what he needs to do his homework (or forget what the assignments are entirely)?
- Does he flit from activity to activity?
- Does he have trouble sticking with chores or other mundane endeavors?
- Does he seem like he's not listening or is off in the clouds?
- Does he have an eternally messy bedroom and backpack?
- Does he have trouble following instructions?

If you answered "yes" to any of these questions, then your child may be struggling with attention symptoms.

Does your child show signs of being hyperactive? Kids with problems in this area can seem like whirling dervishes—they can't sit still, they pick up (and drop) everything in stores, they're chatterboxes, and quiet pursuits rarely keep them entertained.

Is your child impulsive? Children with symptoms of impulsivity are the ones who don't seem to think before they act or speak. They seem not to learn from their mistakes, they interrupt others' conversations, and they have trouble learning to take turns when the other kids do.

A diagnosis of ADHD requires a minimum number of certain symptoms that have lasted for an extended period of time (vs. being a brief phase). If you have observed symptoms of hyperactivity, inattention, or impulsivity in your child for several months, then you may want to adjust your tech rules to protect your child and maximize the benefit she gets out of digital media.

Digital Risks for Hyperactive and Impulsive Children

- Inability to turn off games and the Internet
- Difficulty "changing gears"
- Risk of dangerous impulsive behavior (e.g., sexting, oversharing)
- Greater risk of becoming overstimulated by digital technology
- Greater vulnerability to violent and overstimulating games and movies
- Higher risk of Internet addiction
- Higher risk of problematic usage

Digital Risks for Inattentive and Disorganized Children

- Inability to turn off games and the Internet
- Difficulty "changing gears"
- Increased risk for distraction
- Risk that online behavior will lead to greater disorganization
- Higher risk of Internet addiction
- Higher risk of problematic usage

How can I get my son to turn off the games?

Children with ADHD symptoms have more difficulty unplugging. In a study of video game use among 11- to 12-year-old boys and girls, those children with ADHD had more difficulty getting off their video games than the control group.[1] ADHD stands for "attention-deficit/hyperactivity disorder." The name is a bit of a misnomer since people with ADHD have an abundance of attention but don't regulate it as well as other people. This means that they have trouble shifting attention—a tendency to have "attention deficit" on unpleasant tasks and an overabundance of attention on pleasurable or rewarding tasks. Attention dysregulation is a recipe for disaster when you sprinkle in online games or Internet shopping and surfing. Gaming is particularly problematic for younger children with ADHD.

Neuroscientists have identified the neurotransmitter dopamine as the primary mediator in ADHD. Decreased dopamine in the prefrontal cortex and striatum contribute to inattention, attention dysregulation, and overattention. Decreased levels of dopamine have been linked to both inattention and "overattention" in ADHD. Hyperfocus is a strength when a child matures and can harness it. In children and teenagers, however, it often results in becoming engrossed in TV, games, or the Internet. Normally developing children with moderate technology use do not miss out on other physical and stimulating life activities. But I do find that kids with ADHD can become so engrossed that they "lose time" and miss out on opportunities for real-life play. Their inability to "shut down" and transition creates challenges for parents and caregivers. If only I had a nickel for every parent who has told me that their biggest family conflict was unplugging in the evenings. For parents, it is critical to understand how hard it is for kids who have ADHD to unplug. It is easier for parents to be patient and helpful when they understand that their child is not always being oppositional and defiant but rather struggling to shift gears.

> It is critical to understand how hard it is for kids who have ADHD to unplug.

My Recommendations for Managing Technology and ADHD

✓ Establish clear time limits for game and Internet use.

✓ Use a big timer that is not embedded in a phone or computer.

✓ Start giving warnings 15 minutes prior to shutdown.

✓ Give reminders every 5 minutes prior to shutdown.

✓ Help with the transition by clarifying the next activity.

✓ Provide encouragement when your child is able to unplug successfully.

✓ Recognize that shifting attention and tasks is a learned skill.

Is it possible that my son becomes more hyperactive and violent after playing video games?

Violent video games do not directly cause violence in the real world. People who identify as being "angry" are more likely to become aggressive after playing violent video games. Kids who express anger are more likely to seek out video games with mature (MA) ratings. There is evidence that children use video games to express and work out their anger in a healthy way. Video games can be a good outlet for the safe expression of anger. However, kids who are predisposed to hyperactive and impulsive behavior are at greater risk for becoming agitated or hyperactive after playing highly stimulating or violent games. In my office, parents of elementary- and middle-school-age children with ADHD observe that their children become more agitated or aggressive after extended game use. Fast-paced video games suit the cognitive style of ADHD. They provide an ever-changing, multimodal stimulus and immediate reward with minimal delay.[2] Children with ADHD are more likely to be high energy and impulsive, and more likely to hyperfocus on the game and have trouble shifting attention to something else. Therefore, we often see an increase in agitated behavior after extended game or Internet use. Kids with ADHD are often the first ones in their friend group to play Call of Duty or Mortal Combat. Parents of kids with ADHD need to be extra-vigilant in monitoring the content of games and the quality of their child's online and gaming life.

My Recommendations for Video Games If Your Child Has Symptoms of ADHD

✓ Do not allow MA-rated games.

✓ Add 2 years to manufacturer recommendations.

✓ Understand what types of games your child plays.

✓ Observe your child's behavior after he turns off the computer or game.

✓ Discourage evening play if gaming leads to more agitated behavior.

✓ Reward kids for successfully unplugging or shifting tasks.

Is it possible that my son is addicted to video and online games?

Yes. Children and teenagers with ADHD are at higher risk for Internet and gaming problems and addictions. Internet addiction is not recognized as a disorder in the latest edition of the *Diagnostic and Statistical Manual of Mental Disorders* (DSM-5), meaning that the American medical community has not recognized it as a formal medical or psychiatric disorder. There has been much debate, and I suspect that it will eventually be officially codified. Currently, pathological gambling is the only behavioral addiction officially recognized by the medical community. There are no standardized criteria, so it's difficult to determine prevalence accurately. Internet addiction has been broadly defined as:

■ A preoccupation with the Internet, electronic communication, or games
■ Inability to control usage
■ Distress when unable to use technology

If you're trying to determine whether your child's technology use is problematic, I recommend keeping these guidelines in mind:

■ It is not the duration of usage that matters but the quality of usage.
■ Preoccupation with gaming when not on the game can be a red flag.
■ Distress when unable to use the computer or games is a red flag.
■ Your child's ability to "hyperfocus" on games does not rule out ADHD as a possible diagnosis.
■ Hyperfocus can be a problem if it leads to excessive use or an inability to unplug.

Despite the public debate, we all agree that problematic Internet and video game usage is pervasive. In Asia, they report "addiction" rates as high as 25% in teenagers. There are reports that comorbidity is as high as 30–50%. This means that 30–50% of people with ADHD also suffer from Internet addiction. Attention dysregulation and impulsivity go hand in hand with problematic use of digital technology. In a study of 2,000 adolescents followed over 2 years, the presence of psychiatric symptoms was the strongest predictor for Internet addiction. ADHD topped the list as the single strongest predictor for "Internet addiction."[3] Symptoms associated with ADHD, such as impulsivity, extraversion, disinhibition, and low self-esteem, have also been correlated with problematic Internet use.[4] Kids with ADHD may have a vulnerability to the immediate feedback and a drive to win more coins or get to the next level. Video games have been found to increase the level of dopamine in the brain, further reinforcing problematic usage.

In 2009, an American and South Korean research team studied Internet video game use and ADHD. They concluded that many children with ADHD use Internet video games as a form of self-medication. Video game use has been shown to increase dopamine levels, and ADHD has been linked to decreased dopamine in the striatum and prefrontal cortex. They also found that treating children with Concerta (a long-acting stimulant used for ADHD) led to a decrease in time spent on the Internet and decreased symptoms of Internet addiction.[5] It may be that Internet addiction and ADHD share a common etiology. It seems that the symptoms of ADHD make Internet and video game use very attractive, but the Internet and gaming may worsen symptoms of ADHD.

> Children who have symptoms of ADHD are at higher risk for problematic use of digital technology.

My Recommendations for Managing Problematic Use of Digital Technology

✓ Talk to your kids and teenagers about hyperfocusing.

✓ Help them recognize that they have trouble unplugging.

✓ Help kids and teenagers set reasonable time limits and use timers.

√ Use lots of gentle reminders to prepare them for unplugging. Encourage healthy use.

√ Take breaks when use becomes unhealthy.

Is my teenager who has ADHD safe on social media?

Teens and tweens with impulsivity are at risk for problematic use of social media, electronic communication, and the Internet. The anonymity and pace of technology make everyone a little bit more impulsive. For most people, a little bit of impulsivity is not a problem. However, if you are prone to impulsive behavior, you can get into a lot of trouble very quickly. Snapchat and Ask.fm are two of the biggest areas of concern. On Snapchat, you send a picture and set how long it will last, from 0 to 10 seconds, before "disappearing." However, the recipient can easily save the picture by taking a screenshot. The sender is notified when a screenshot is taken. Ask.fm is an anonymous question-asking platform. It has become a notorious breeding ground for hate speech and bullying. Teens with ADHD are more likely to post an inappropriate picture or make an impulsive comment. Teenagers with ADHD need to be aware of their symptoms. They need to take their time when posting or responding. They should consider getting friends or family to look at comments or pictures prior to posting. If they are mindful of their symptoms, then they can take a thoughtful approach to social media.

> Make your teen with ADHD aware of her symptoms so she'll understand why you encourage her to take her time when posting or responding on social media.

Disorganized Children and Teenagers

Teddy is an 11-year-old sixth grader who was referred to me because he is distracted and getting a C in English. I ask him about his homework, and he says that he does it but forgets to turn it in. I ask him if he checks his backpack at night, and he rolls his eyes at me. He explains that he e-mails the homework to his teacher. If that is the case, I ask, then how does he forget it? He opens his laptop and shows me the 60 folders that are open on his desktop and explains that he knows he did it but can't find it.

Should my child use traditional organization tools or technology for organization and planning?

Technology both solves and creates challenges in organization. People with ADHD struggle with organization and executive planning (the ability to plan ahead). Technology should be used as a tool for organizing and planning ahead. Organization and executive planning must be taught just like algebra and chemistry. Many organizational coaches will recommend paper calendars and assignment books for kids. As a digital immigrant, I understand the appeal of the visual poster board calendar and the easily flippable homework pad. Digital natives are as comfortable on apps as they are with wire-bound notebooks. The goal is to help your child or teen develop a consistent system that helps him organize homework and plan ahead for papers, tests, and social events.

My Recommendations
for Helping a Child or Teen Get Organized

✓ **Step 1** is the big calendar. Executive planning isn't fully developed until college. Even your teenager needs help in planning ahead. He needs a big-picture visual of his week and month. I no longer recommend the wall calendar to tweens. I prefer the apps such as Corkulous, which allows you to make your own corkboard with notes, pictures, lists, and calendars.

✓ **Step 2** is the homework planner. The iHomework app allows you to keep track of assignments. Any system works as long as all homework is in one place and there is a section for long-term assignments. Check with your tween or teen's school to find out where, when, and whether homework and tests are posted online.

✓ **Step 3** is taking notes. Kids with ADHD are notoriously poor note takers. Evernote is a very popular app that allows you to organize and take class notes. You can record audio notes and insert pictures. Also check with your child's school to see if teachers hand out or post copies of class notes.

✓ **Step 4** is setting priorities. Priority Matrix helps teenagers assess the short-term and long-term importance of multiple assignments. Teens need a daily and weekly game plan for homework. Teenagers often make the mistake of spending too much time on unimportant assignments and neglecting critical work.

√ **Step 5** is managing time. I continue to recommend an old-fashioned oven timer. I don't like the iPhone for timers. It is an excuse to pick up the phone that you don't need at the moment. Help your tween or teen keep track of the time it takes for each assignment and assess efficiency.

√ **Step 6** is social life. The goal is to balance work and play. If your teen's calendar has only academic due dates, then she can't plan her whole life. If your son has a basketball game the night before a big chemistry test, he needs to study in advance. Your teen or tween's whole life should be visible on one calendar. Google calendar is the easiest calendar, and parents can send invites to events and appointments that they schedule. Galndr (name rhymes with *calendar*) is a new calendar app designed for teenage girls. It is pink and allows girls to have private and public events and inner circles for their BFFs. It has stricter privacy settings than Facebook. Kids need to be wary of privacy settings when posting schedules on social media. The entire world does not need to know that your teenage son is on a class trip to Washington, D.C.

SOCIAL ANXIETY AND POOR SOCIAL SKILLS

David is a 17-year-old 12th grader sent to see me because he is "depressed." His parents report that he rarely leaves his room and is on his computer 24/7. They say he is very bright and attends a gifted high school. However, he is tired all the time and interested only in being online. His parents are concerned that he is depressed and addicted to the Internet. When I meet him, he is a bit disheveled and makes minimal eye contact. He is socially awkward but warms up after a few minutes. I ask him about his life online. I ask him if he knows anything about coding and building games. He looks up and seems a bit intrigued by the question. He goes into a detailed explanation of how to build a game. He tells me that he is building a game with his best friend. This time I perk up and ask him about the "best friend." He says that she is 20 years old and lives in Seattle (he lives in Connecticut). They are collaborating on his new project. The time change has posed some challenges, but he is excited about the multiplayer game they are building. He tells me that he has two friends at school that he sits with at lunch. They talk about games and technology. He doesn't see them out of school but is in contact with them through texts and games. He is collaborating with one of them on a robotics project. He admits that he is not that "social" and becomes anxious with real-life interactions. He is irritated with his parents' nagging. He denies being depressed or having difficulty with sleep.

David's story represents what is so confusing about adolescent online interactions. David is not social and not that interested in making friends. He might have met criteria for what used to be called Asperger syndrome. Asperger syndrome is no longer officially recognized by the medical and psychiatric community. David is a little bit different from his peers, and his real-life social skills are not fluid. Digital technology is a double-edged sword for him. He uses the Internet to connect with other people worldwide who share his interest in building games. He is a very accomplished coder and gamer. He has "colleagues" and "collaborators" online who respect him and want to work with him. In school he does not have close friends, but he is not depressed. He does avoid real interactions when he spends all day and night online. His family has encouraged him to connect online with classmates with whom he shares interests. Some teenagers like David build self-esteem and confidence from online connections. However, David's online skills do not always generalize to real-life social interactions. David's challenge is to safely enjoy and connect online while not abandoning real-life relationships and experiences.

Parents need to help their socially avoidant kids to connect online. There is no reason for kids with pervasive developmental disorders (high-functioning autism spectrum) or simply poor social skills to remain isolated. Isolated children and teenagers may be able to find their voice on the Internet. There are also lots of opportunities to cultivate computer and technology skills. Many young adults with high-functioning pervasive developmental disorders attend school and work in jobs that they can do via the Internet. Of course, you want to maximize your child or teenager's social skills as he or she is growing up. The key is to help your child find healthy outlets online and to be aware of how your

> Socially awkward and anxious teenagers often turn to online relationships to avoid real-life interactions.

teenager is using the Internet. If you know that your teenager struggles with social interactions, then you need to be wary about and involved in how he spends his time online.

> **Is it possible that my daughter prefers social media and texting to real-life interactions?**

Most healthy teenagers prefer face-to-face interactions but find electronic communication and social media to be more convenient. Children and teenagers with social anxiety may use digital technology as an escape from their real lives.

Social anxiety disorder involves the extreme fear of being scrutinized and judged by others in social or performance situations. It can wreak havoc on the lives of those who suffer from it. Social anxiety disorder goes beyond shyness. There is a heightened self-consciousness and fear of scrutiny in social situations. The typical age of onset is 13 years. Social anxiety disorder is an official psychiatric disorder with criteria and duration requirements. Once again, I am less concerned with whether your teenager or tween meets specific criteria. I do worry about children and teens who are excessively self-conscious in social situations.

Social anxiety is a risk factor for problematic digital technology use. Teens who are socially anxious often turn to the Internet and social media for social connectedness because of their fear of face-to-face interactions. Socially anxious teenagers prefer online disclosure to offline disclosure.[6] It is wonderful when they can connect and build confidence online. A challenge for socially anxious teenagers is to present their real self online. They are often concerned that no one will like their real self, so they present a false or "fake" self. Researchers have found that those who "fake" it online are more likely to suffer from anxiety and poor social skills.[7] I believe that online connections are more likely to generalize to real-life skills if the teenager is able to present her real self in cyberspace.

Socially anxious teens have much more at stake on the Internet. They are more likely to become overly dependent on online connections and relationships. Socially anxious teens report that Facebook support contributes to their sense of well-being beyond face-to-face support. Nonanxious individuals do not report that social media connections contribute to their well-being.[8] There is a risk that digital technology will feed avoidance and worsen fears of real-life interactions.[9] There is concern that teenagers who are overly dependent on the Internet and prefer online disclosure may be more vulnerable to online predators. The pros and cons of digital technology need to be weighed carefully. Parents need to take an active role in helping socially anxious kids find confidence and support online that can be generalized to their real lives.

> Social anxiety is a risk factor for problematic Internet usage.

My Recommendations for Digital Technology Use by Socially Anxious Children and Teens

✓ Help your teenager present his or her real self on social media and the Internet.

✓ If your teenager is socially awkward, encourage him to use the Internet for self-expression and social connectedness.

✓ Be wary if your teenager becomes overly involved with one person online.

✓ Help your socially awkward child cultivate both digital and real-life relationships.

✓ Encourage your anxious child or teen to connect to real-life friends and classmates via texts and social media.

✓ Encourage online disclosure in moderation.

✓ If online interactions are making your child anxious, take a break.

✓ Be wary of overdependence or excessive reassurance seeking online.

✓ Be aware of whether online interactions are replacing real-life interactions.

✓ Be wary of teenagers who are preoccupied with online relationships and who are distressed when they are unable to connect online.

✓ Help anxious tweens or teens not to disclose personal information or make plans to meet strangers.

DEPRESSION, SUICIDE, AND DIGITAL MEDIA

Nadia, an 18-year-old depressed teenager from Ontario, had three exchanges with "Cami," a 31-year-old depressed nurse, in a suicide chat room in 2005. "Cami" suggested that Nadia hang herself rather than drown herself. She even suggested what type of rope to use. Cami offered to guide Nadia through the process via a webcam. After her chat with "Cami," Nadia chose to jump off a bridge. Local authorities found her body 1 month later. "Cami" turned out to be a 45-year-old man named William Melchert-Dinkel, who has been convicted of two counts of assisted suicide and admitted to encouraging dozens of depressed people to commit suicide.

Jessica Laney was a 16-year-old girl who hung herself after being bullied on the question-and-answer social media site Ask.fm. She was called "fat" and a "slut," and one person posted, "Can you kill yourself already?" According to her Ask.fm posts, she struggled with family issues, school conflict, and concerns about her body image. She sought support on social media and found abuse instead.

Admittedly, I have chosen two extreme examples of teenage suicide that are linked to digital technology. The statistics on suicide and depression make this a group that we must address as we carve out our digital blueprint.

- **Suicide is the third leading cause of death for 15- to 24-year-olds.**
- **11% of young people suffer from depression by the age of 18.**
- **Depression is the leading cause of disability worldwide for 15- to 44-year-olds.**[10]

Digital technology does not cause or worsen depression. In fact, there may be ways for technology to be a tool for screening and prevention. As a parent, you need to be on guard for depression. Your teenager's technology use may offer you a way to identify depression and intervene. I am not so concerned that technology causes depression. Adolescent depression existed well before the first computer was invented. Teenagers who are depressed are certainly more vulnerable to online predators and cyberbullying. If your teenager is depressed, then you should be monitoring for cyberbullying, online predators, and visits to dangerous pro-suicide websites.

The Invisible-Risk Group

My big concern is that most parents don't recognize when their adolescents become depressed. It can be hard to tease out normal teenager irritability and oppositionality from depression. **Parents have a tendency to blame gaming and social media when technology use is usually a symptom, not the cause.** In a European study by the Saving and Empowering Young Lives in Europe (SEYLE) organization, 12,000 adolescents were divided into three groups:

■ High-risk group (13%): higher rates of alcohol, drug, and cigarette use and truancy
■ Low-risk group (58%): low rates of alcohol, drug, and cigarette use; low rates of truancy and Internet use; more time spent sleeping and exercising
■ Invisible-risk group (27%): higher rates of Internet use and less time sleeping and exercising

No one is surprised that the teens who exhibited risky behaviors fell into the "high-risk" group for mental health problems. We didn't need a 12,000-person study to give us that finding. What might surprise you is that the "invisible-risk" group's rates of depression, anxiety, and suicidal thoughts were similar to those of the "high-risk" group.[11]

Depressed teenagers and adults have different patterns of Internet usage. Teens who play games and use the Internet for more than 5 hours per day may be at higher risk for sadness, suicidal ideation, and suicidal planning but not for suicide attempts, according to a survey done in 2007 and 2009.[12] The online activities of 216 participating undergraduates at Missouri University of Science and Technology were monitored, and the findings showed consistent patterns of use.

Depressed college students were found to be more likely to:

■ Spend more time on the Internet.
■ Send more e-mail messages.

- Use the Internet in a random way with lots of switching between games, video, and communication.
- Spend more time watching videos, playing games, and chatting.[13]

Sriram Chellappan, the lead researcher, explained, "We believe that your pattern of Internet use says something about you. Specifically, our research suggests it can offer clues to your mental well-being." The social media world is becoming increasingly aware of how people may turn to social media when they are feeling depressed and suicidal. Facebook has launched an antisuicide initiative. It has partnered with the National Suicide Prevention Lifeline and SAVE, a national suicide prevention organization. Facebook friends can report people they are concerned about. Suicide counselors will contact flagged people. Facebook is also working on an initiative to identify high-risk users by looking for problematic patterns and keywords. In 2012, researchers looked at 1.7 million tweets by 1.2 million users from May to August. They compared rates of suicide comments on Twitter with actual rates of suicide in a particular state. The suicide tweets correlated with the rates of suicide. Midwestern states, western states, and Alaska had a higher proportion of suicide-related tweeters. Twitter has the potential to serve as a tool for real-time monitoring of suicide risk factors and a platform for intervention. Right now, parents can monitor their teenagers' social media and texts for depression and suicide content.

Can the Internet serve as support for my depressed teen?

Yes. The Internet, social media, and some online games can provide support. Suicides have been prevented and depressions treated when an online friend reaches out and gets real-life support. There is plenty of good information about depression online that can lead teenagers to hotlines and help. Unfortunately, teenagers who go looking for help can easily find themselves on pro-suicide or pro-self-harm sites. You can order suicide kits and copies of *Final Exit*, the pro-suicide movement's bible. Researchers have found that watching suicide videos and going to suicide sites increased the risk of actual suicide. Most teenagers who have attempted suicide admit to looking online for ideas and informa-tion.[14]

The biggest mistake that a parent can make is to take away the phone and the computer of a depressed adolescent. You may further your teenager's isolation and take away his or her only supports. Recently, I worked with a high school student who was being bullied at school. At home, she was irritable, argumentative, and always on her phone. Her parents were worried that she was depressed and were annoyed by her stubborn and argumentative behavior. They felt that there should be "consequences" for her bad behavior. So they took away her phone. When we explored it further, it turned out that her phone was a lifeline and critical support for her. She texted her mother from school when she was lonely. She called or messaged her friends outside of school to find reassurance and support. Without her phone, she was stuck with the "mean girls" at school and felt unsupported. The family and I recognized that she was depressed, and we initiated family and individual therapy. She kept the phone, and her parents used other "conse-quences" to deal with her oppositional behav-ior. Over time the depression and bullying improved. Her attachment to her phone became more reasonable and less frantic. Sometimes it is appropriate and necessary to not take away the phone.

> Parents need to understand how their teenagers use the phone and the Internet before they take either away.

The take-home point is to look for red flags for depression and recognize when technology use is problematic. Digital technology in moderation is an integral and positive component of high school. However, children who are depressed or anxious join the "invisible-risk" group.

As noted above, it's not always easy to know when a teen is depressed. Children and teens with depression often don't fit the clas-sic picture of acting down and dejected but may be more likely to act irritated and angry. If your child *is* often sad, expresses hopelessness, seems oversensitive to criticism, or feels guilty, talk to your pediatri-cian. A depressed child or teen may also seem bored and uninterested in former hobbies, or complain of being tired or having a lot of stom-achaches or headaches. Depression can cause problems with sleeping and changes in eating habits. Relationships may become difficult, the child may avoid school, and grades might fall. Ask your teenager if he has thoughts about killing himself or dying. Teenagers rarely offer this information but may answer you honestly if asked directly. If your child expresses any suicidal thoughts or exhibits any of the symptoms above for longer than a week, then definitely seek help from your pediatrician or a mental health professional.

WORRISOME TECHNOLOGY PATTERNS

- Abrupt change in how the child uses the Internet, social media, and games
- Erratic use of the Internet with lots of switching
- Dramatic increase in electronic communication
- Overdependence on a single online relationship
- Avoidance of school or friends to stay online
- Significant sleep impairment from online activities
- Browser history that shows visits to suicide or self-harm sites
- Worrisome posts or pictures on social media sites
- Cyberbullying

What to Do If You're Worried about Depression and Problematic Technology Usage

✓ Talk to your child or teenager.

✓ Ask directly about hopelessness, self-harm, and suicide.

✓ If he won't talk to you, then find someone he will talk to.

✓ Inquire in a **noncritical** way about what the child or teen is doing online.

✓ Take an interest in the child's online activities.

✓ Find out how technology is supportive and helpful for your teen or child.

✓ Inquire about cyberbullying.

✓ Check the browser history.

✓ Check the phone.

✓ Check the child or teen's social media posts.

✓ Google your teenager.

✓ Set limits around sleep and technology.

✓ Inquire about drugs and alcohol.

✓ **Get professional help if symptoms don't improve.**

Digital technology can be a powerful tool to help increase efficiency for those with ADHD and provide critical support and intervention for anxious and depressed kids. It's important to understand your children's challenges with attention, distractibility, and anxiety, and look for changes in behavior that might signal depression. If you are concerned about your child or teenager, then you must be accommodating, flexible, and vigilant as you customize your family technology rules in the next chapter.

> Parents who have lost a child to suicide regret "respecting" their child's privacy. Monitoring your child's digital life could save his real life.

12 Don't Take Away the Phone!

The Nuts and Bolts of Your Family Digital Technology Agreement

Katrina is the resident sixth-grade hacker in her middle school. Other kids pay her $20 per "jailbreak." She hacks into their games and instantaneously they have thousands of coins or gems. She has a Twitter account that her parents don't know about and a fake Instagram account that her parents think she uses. Her parents don't have any of her passwords. When they figure out how to delete violent games and apps, she immediately reloads them. They often take away her phone, but she uses her school-issued Android tablet. She has impersonated a friend or acquaintance online and caused drama in her social circles. Her parents are very loving but very busy and not on the same page at all. They come down hard with lots of rules but don't enforce them. One parent says one thing and the other parent says another. Katrina is always one step ahead of them. She wants her parents' approval and attention badly. She does not meet criteria for an Internet addiction. She has lots of other interests. She plays basketball and participates in every school play. She is happy to be off with friends without the Internet or her phone. She isn't sexting. For Katrina, it is an issue of control with her parents. As they say in the celebrity world, negative attention is better than no attention at all.

The take-home points here are:

- Emphasize consistency over quantity of rules.
- When it comes to establishing rules, the younger the better (Katrina's parents are playing catch-up).
- Be on the same page as your child's other parent (or at least fake it).
- Make rules simple and manageable.
- Don't sweat the small stuff.

It is finally time to write a family agreement that reflects your family's values, priorities, and realities. My goal is to help you start the dialogue with your spouse and your kids on the technology stuff that matters. Forget about the perfect points/rewards/stickers/coupons. Not the goal here!

Your family plan can be broken down into the five W's:

- When
- Where
- What
- Who
- What if

INTRODUCTION TO THE BEHAVIORAL PLAN

Behavioral plans are the trickiest aspect of being a child and adolescent psychiatrist or therapist. When I am teaching young doctors and psychologists, I warn them about the pitfalls of the "star chart." Well-meaning parents and teachers set up complicated systems with stars, stickers, coupons, tokens, coins, and candy. Sometimes they work temporarily, but they rarely translate into long-term internalized change. In my experience, they rarely get started.

A social worker I work with runs a parenting group. She orders bulk pirate coins and stickers from Oriental Trading to give to parents in her group. She has found that many busy parents never even get the stickers or coins needed to initiate the plan. Additionally, the parents who need the behavior charts the most are the ones least likely to follow through. It is very demoralizing to get a sticker chart going and not be able to follow through.

I want your children and teenagers to know that there are guidelines and rules regarding digital technology. I want them to internalize the ethics of digital citizenship. Your agreement should emphasize behavioral expectations and not get lost in the details. Recently I consulted with the mom of a 7-year-old boy with ADHD. I was so impressed with all of her charts. She gave out 30-minute media coupons and took them away when the child misbehaved. She was organized and had a thoughtful system. I asked her how it was going. She explained that her son brushes his teeth and does his homework now, but he spends all day fighting with her about the coupons.

I started *Screen-Smart Parenting* talking about parenting styles and parents' relationship with technology. I am concluding the book with these two topics. Parents need to be honest with themselves about who they are when trying to develop a plan for technology. I will use myself as an example. We are a media-moderate family, and I have a permissive/authoritative parenting style. My husband has a more authoritative style that I often envy. My children haven't exhibited any red flags for problematic Internet usage, but my oldest child is only 9 years old, so there is still time.

I admit it. I love to set up beautiful behavioral plans that I can't maintain for more than a few days. My children recognize my lack of follow-through and remind me about the rewards that I "owe" them. My husband and I have full-time jobs and we lead busy lives. We have wonderful caregivers, but we are outnumbered with three children and can't monitor everything. We value technology and want our children to be screen-smart but use technology wisely.

We use an organic task–reward model for technology during the week. This means that homework, playdates, and soccer practice come first and Angry Birds comes later. My 9-year-old talks about safe boundaries online and is willing to read books if packaged in iPad wrapping paper. My 7-year-old knows that he must be kind online, and my 5-year-old is rushing to learn her letters so she can type on our Bluetooth iPad keyboards like her brothers. Is it perfect? No. There are parents with more balanced authoritative styles, more time, and fewer children who do it much better than us. At this moment, there is too much Doc McStuffins, Clash of Clans, and MyNBA2K14 for my taste. My husband and I use our iPhones too much. My children know that we are constantly struggling to find a balance and to find new educational ways to use technology. I want them to know that there are guidelines and restrictions and that we all struggle to find a balance. I want them to be mindful that they will be struggling to maintain this balance throughout their lives. It is not perfect, but it is thoughtful and mirrors who we are.

> Our children should know that they will be struggling with maintaining balance in the use of technology throughout their lives.

Behavioral Chart Recommendations and Realities

✓ Prioritize your goals.

✓ Keep goals and expectations realistic.

✓ Develop a plan that is easy to achieve.

✓ Organic, short-term rewards are most successful.

✓ Avoid long-term, expensive rewards.

✓ Make expectations very simple and concrete.

✓ Don't leave criteria open to debate.

✓ Build in end points.

✓ Remember that the goal is to internalize behavior so reward charts are no longer needed.

I want to elaborate on some of the details above and apply them to technology. Pick the detail that you care about the most and develop behavioral expectations around it. My children don't love to read, and that bothers me. I am less concerned about whether they play an interactive Wii game with their friends. I don't want them to play Clash of Clans to the exclusion of reading. However, if they want to play educational or reading games on their iPad, then I don't want to restrict them. Parents of tweens and teens may be concerned about grades and friends. I have heard parents say to me that if their teenager continues to make good grades they don't need to "police" the amount of time the teen spends on the Internet. The goal of our agreement is to set forth both behavioral and ethical expectations. If you spend their childhood fighting over 15-minute increments, you may lose the broader battle of creating an open dialogue where your child can become a caring and creative digital citizen.

Ask any behaviorist about reinforcement and you will hear that positive reinforcement is more likely to be internalized than negative reinforcement. Basically, punishment may stop a behavior in the moment, but fear doesn't always translate into long-term change. The best rewards are naturally built in and use a positive reinforcement model. For example, if you get ready for school first, then you can use the remaining time to play on your phone or iPad. If you are going to attempt a behavioral plan, the criteria must be argument-proof. Criteria can't be "behave" or "be good." Define "good" or "behave." Criteria must be concrete and measurable, such as "get dressed" before using the iPad or "finish all assignments due the next day" prior to logging on to social media.

Lastly, it is content, not quantity, that matters. Over and over again, the research finds that it is content you need to be worried about. My agreement will broadly outline timing and location, but I want to emphasize that content and the way technology is used are what matters.

> **A behavioral plan has to be based on criteria that are argument-proof.**

WHEN?

"When?" and "How long?" are the million-dollar questions for parents with kids under 12 years. Parents of older kids do worry about time spent, but habits are hard to break. Parents of tweens and teens are rightfully focused on their children's safety, privacy, and balance. Three questions that I often hear are:

"Should my children use technology during the week?"

"How much time should they be allowed to use technology?"

"Which types of technology or devices should they use at each age?"

We covered question 3 in Part II. We've also discussed questions 1 and 2, but now you have to make a decision. The AAP recommends no more than 2 hours per day of technology. Two hours is a far cry from the reality, which ranges from 4 to 12 hours depending on age. My recommendation is to deemphasize time limits and focus on content and safety.

Should my child use technology during the week?

I know that most readers want a firm answer to this question, but I must hedge on the weekday question. It is OK for children to use technology during the week, but it is a personal choice that parents must make. If you can restrict during the week without creating conflict and without pushing your children underground, then go for it. If TV and games are part of the weekday routine, then make it work. If you allow technology during the week, there should be clear guidelines. I encourage doing required tasks first and then "earning" TV and game time afterward. Trying to get kids off the TV and games to start homework can be challenging. By the time your child gets a smartphone, the weekday restrictions are gone. Your tween will begin to use technology in the way most adults use it. He will use it in the classroom and throughout the day in some way. At that point, the discussion turns more toward balance and less toward restrictions.

How much time should they be allowed to use technology?

Again, these numbers depend on whether you are a media-light, media-moderate, or media-heavy family. I can give you some guidelines. I suggest that you don't get caught up in exact times with younger kids. Media may be part of your child's life but should not drive it.

General Recommendations for Tech Time

✓ Don't give exact times for children under 8 years. (They don't have an adult's sense of time.)

✓ You can use TV episodes as a timer for young kids, for example, one short show (15 minutes) or two long shows (60 minutes).

✓ Use pictures and cartoons for schedules with younger children.

✓ Err on the side of play, but there are lots of educational technology opportunities for younger children.

✓ Required activities, chores, and homework should be done prior to technology use.

✓ From Sunday to Thursday, I recommend a 30- to 90-minute technology-free homework period. This is time for homework that does not need to be done on the computer or tablet. If computers are required, then make it a phone-free time.

✓ Instead of fighting over duration of play, give clear departure times and bedtimes. For instance, technology turned off at 9:30 P.M. for sleep and 7:30 A.M. for school.

✓ Be wary of kids rushing through work to get online. If that happens, have an adult review homework before giving back the phone or letting the child go online.

✓ Distraction is the best way to build a life for your child that is not media heavy. Children report watching TV and going online when they are bored. You can't entertain your children all the time, but if they have after-school programs and playdates, then they may have less reason and less time to end up on technology.

✓ Take the tech-free challenge and find 30 minutes each day where the entire family unplugs. Perhaps your family can't find that 30 minutes daily; then try for a few times per week. The tech-free challenge sends a powerful message that the entire family is trying to find time to unplug together.

✓ If your child has had a full technology-free day, there may be nothing wrong with relaxing with TV or a game in the evening.

✓ If you are concerned about a tween or teenager's Internet use at night, then turn off the Internet at your home at a certain time in the evening.

✓ Remember that children and teenagers should unplug 30 minutes prior to bedtime.

WHERE?

"Where" is the easiest part of this equation. In the pre-smartphone ages (0–around 11), there should be no computers, iPads, or gaming consoles in bedrooms. When you are building the foundation for your family's digital technology use, try using technology in common areas, whether it is a kitchen, den, or playroom. I would prefer young kids who do use technology for homework to always use it in a common room. It builds a habit of using technology where there is supervision and assistance.

I encourage communal "charging stations" in common areas. Parents and kids can get in the habit of leaving their devices to charge elsewhere. The communal charging stations help tweens and teens to part with their phones at night. The goal is to eliminate texts or messages from popping up throughout the night.

> Homework done with technology should be done in a common room.

Parents often complain about the car. You do need guidelines for technology in the car. These guidelines will be specific to your family's needs. Many families don't allow technology in the car on a daily basis but make exceptions for long school bus rides or an extended carpool trip. There are inherent risks to using technology on the school bus. Your child may be with older kids and won't be monitored. I recommend that younger children do not go online or use devices with 3G capabilities when on an unsupervised bus ride. If your tween does have a smartphone or tablet with 3G capabilities, check the browser history after the ride. Many parents who drive carpools want to talk to their kids or want their kids to talk to each other. I don't recommend technology on a daily basis in the car. I would allow it if you have a child who is sitting in a carpool line for 30 minutes or spends his afternoon in a car that is shuttling siblings around. In that case, I would pick educational games and videos and encourage occasional breaks.

Young children shouldn't use 3G devices while on unsupervised bus rides.

Texting and driving is a national epidemic. We all know it, but I would be remiss not to include it in this section. Most teenagers have seen a parent talk or text while driving. Teenagers should not be on the phone when they are driving. I would set clear limits and check phone history if necessary. Teenagers should use a car GPS and not a smartphone navigation app. They should pull over if they need to contact their parents, and they should not pick up friends' calls or texts while driving. There are lots of rules about driving, so voice call and texting rules should be seamlessly included.

WHAT?

The content is what matters. All content is not created equal. Brain Quest, Tangrams, Stack the States, and Words with Friends are quality educational games. Clash of Clans, Temple Run, Grand Theft Auto, and Mortal Combat have less value. Your kids must become your partners in figuring out what is appropriate. I always ask my older children what is appropriate for my younger ones. My 9-year-old son has begun to build a vocabulary he can use to explain why someone might or might not like a certain game. I would encourage your kids to write "reviews" of games, apps, and websites that they like or want. The goal is to raise critical consumers who can make good choices for themselves.

"Technology is a tool" is the mantra that needs to come across as you decorate your children's digital landscape. Tablets and computers can be a tool for reading and academic assistance. A smartphone can be used to text your parents and make plans with your friends. It should not be used to avoid your life or watch inappropriate stuff. You and your children will have to join forces to find **balance**. The technology

I'll say it again: technology is a tool.

agreement applies to adults as well. If parents strike a balance, then it will be easier for children to follow suit.

WHO?

"Who" is the most important part of the family agreement. Who do you want to be online? How can technology cultivate, consolidate, and showcase your child's emerging identity? The essence of raising kids in the 21st century is understanding the depth of **digital citizenship**. The great power of parenting is that you play a huge role in shaping your child's identity. The digital world will provide a ubiquitous tool that they can use or abuse as they grow up. We have reviewed the tenets of digital citizenship, but they need to be spelled out simply in the agreement. Let me be clear. It is not easy to enforce citizenship in your agreement. The tenets need to be in the agreement because your children need to clearly understand what you expect from them. You can't control every choice that they make, but you can give them a foundation to build upon.

Who are you online?

- Smart
- Kind
- Empathetic
- Funny
- Creative
- Socially conscious
- Friendly (but not too flirty)
- Upstanding
- Your best self
- Your hopeful or ideal self
- Your true self

Ask your kids to give examples of each and to add to the list. . . .

WHAT IF?

> **When should I take my child's phone away?**

This may be the most important question and the most commonly asked question in the book. The smartphone has become an incredibly powerful tool for parents. Smartphones are appendages for many tweens and teens. Parents of tweens and teens report lots of conflict around the phone. I am not sure what the phone equivalent was for those of us growing up in the 1960s, '70s, '80s, and early '90s. Even the idea of taking it away strikes fear in the hearts of millennials. Parents have great power and must wield it wisely.

Consequences are the hardest part of this family agreement. It is easier to create a beautiful document that reflects your values and attitudes about digital technology. It is much more difficult to set up real-life consequences that you and your spouse and other caregivers will execute. There are two types of infractions. The first is a time or place infraction, and the second is a content infraction.

Time or Place Infraction

If you allow your children and teens to use technology when it is an appropriate time, they are less likely to have time infractions. The more restrictions you impose, the more your child may eventually go underground. There must be limitations, but we want to avoid sneaky or deceitful use. If you find that your child is sneaking technology, talk to him. Find out what your child thinks is reasonable. Don't feel compelled to follow an 8-year-old's suggestions, but do understand his thought process.

If he uses technology when he is not allowed, then you can dock time from when he is allowed. Don't start out draconian. Set up a weekly plan. For a first infraction, he loses Saturday morning or Friday night use. On the second infraction, he may lose technology privileges for 1 or 2 days. Consequences should start over weekly. I want to caution parents here. If your child is constantly using games and TV when you don't allow it, make sure your agreement is thoughtful. For instance, if he is playing his sports and doing his homework and wants to play Minecraft for 30 minutes in creative mode, then what is your reasoning in not allowing it? If there is a good reason, explain it to him. Remember that the agreement needs to make sense because we want your child to internalize it. Before long, you will lose control and you want him to have the skills to balance his desire for technology with the rest of his life.

Content Infraction

Content infractions are a different issue. Honestly, I am not so concerned about time infractions. My concern is about content infractions. Examples of content infractions include:

- Sending a mean text
- Posting an embarrassing picture of a friend
- Visiting sites repeatedly that are racist, sexist, or homophobic
- Presenting yourself as overly tough or overly sexualized
- Taking credit for others' work
- Getting involved in an online scam
- Connecting with strangers online
- Giving out personal information online
- Agreeing to meet an online "friend" in person
- Downloading or buying MA-rated games
- Stealing or sharing passwords
- Buying or selling drugs or alcohol online

Most parents reading this book would be appalled by any of these infractions. The challenge is to keep the dialogue open enough that you know about the infractions but monitored enough that your teenager can't get away with them for long. In the case of content infractions, I believe in the motto that "the punishment should fit the crime." Yes, you can take away their phone and tablet. But let's be real, most teenagers need a computer for homework and can access the Internet at school or at friends' homes. Take away the devices for a period of time, but make the punishment truly fit the crime if you want it to be meaningful. For example, if your child is bullying or being mean, then he needs to write an apology letter. He needs to make an effort to be kind whether that means volunteering at school or going out of his way to help a classmate in need. If he is buying or selling drugs or alcohol, he should attend an AA meeting and learn about what happens to people who abuse drugs and alcohol.

Turn the infraction into teachable moments. Be aware of when infractions are actually cries for help. Actions speak louder than words. If your child is plagiarizing or stealing work online, you should ask whether he is struggling in school. Does he need more support? Is he in the wrong academic setting? Is there too much academic stress? Each infraction will give you information about what is going on with your child. You can take away the phone, but you also need to solve the problem while you still have the power to do so.

The parents of 61% of teens report that they have rules for the Internet, but only 38% of those teens agree that they have rules. Parents need to find time to sit down and agree on the basic guidelines for technology. At the end of the chapter I present three templates for family digital technology agreements: one each for elementary school, middle school, and high school students. You will obviously need to modify the plan to match your family's needs.

> You can take away the phone, but you also need to solve the problem while you still have the power to do so.

The first step is to sit down with your partner and figure out where you stand. If you're not on exactly the same page, you have to find a compromise and support each other. Of course, divorced parents will presumably have the most challenges here. Ideally, all parents and stepparents involved with implementing this plan will be somewhat involved in creating it. Your teens should not be able to play her parents against each other. I would go as far as to say that parents who can't communicate with each other should employ a parent coach or mediator to draft a family agreement. Once you are on the same page you can sit down with your kids and present the plan. I suggest that you use these templates as a starting point and ask your children to weigh in on each component. They should feel a part of this process, and you should listen to them. In the case of technology, they may know more about it and understand it in a different way.

> Listen to and learn from your tech-savvy kids.

Take the following quiz to help put together your family agreement:

When

1. Will you allow technology during the week? Yes or No. If no, skip to #4.

2. Will you allow technology in the mornings before school? Yes or No

3. If yes, what tasks need to be completed prior to technology use? Circle all that apply.
   a. Wake up and get dressed
   b. Eat breakfast
   c. Brush teeth
   d. Gather belongings and put on coats
   e. Other _____
   f. All of the above

4. Will you allow technology after school? Yes or No

5. If yes, what tasks need to be completed prior to use? Circle all that apply.
   a. After-school activities/sports
   b. Playdates
   c. Homework
   d. Chores
   e. Dinner
   f. Other _____
   g. All of the above

6. At what time should devices be turned off at night? *(recommend 30 minutes prior to bedtime)* _____

Where

7. Is technology allowed in the car? Yes or No

8. If yes, what type of technology? _____

9. Is there a minimum car ride time before technology is allowed? Yes or No

10. If yes, what time? _____ *(would suggest over 20 or 30 minutes)*

11. Is technology allowed on bus rides? Yes, No, or N/A

12. If yes, what type of technology? _____

13. Are computers, tablets, phones, gaming consoles allowed in the bedroom? Yes or No *(Just say NO!)*

14. If yes, at what time should devices be turned off? Time _____

15. Where should technology be placed when sleeping? Choose from the following:
    a. Communal charging station
    b. Parent's bedroom
    c. Other _____

What

16. Are you using any parental controls? Yes or No

17. If yes, list controls. _____

18. If no, how are you monitoring your children's use? Circle all that apply.
    a. Adults use technology with child *(applicable only for young child)*
    b. All technology in common areas
    c. Check browser history
    d. Periodically check tween/teen's texts, phone
    e. Follow tween/teen on social media sites
    f. Periodically have tween/teen show me what he or she is doing online
    g. Permission needed to download apps, games
    h. Tweens/teens need permission to join social media sites, multiplayer games, role-playing games, etc.
    i. Other _____

19. Do you have all of your children's passwords? Yes or No

20. If no, agreement requires that children give parents all passwords for devices, websites, games, and social media sites.

21. What types of games is your child allowed to play? Circle all that apply.

   a. Child must follow ratings.

   b. We use Common Sense Media ratings.

   c. I read reviews before allowing my child to download or buy games.

   d. I ask friends or teachers before allowing game purchases.

   e. I ask my child to explain why he wants a game and to consider the pros and cons of the particular game.

Who

22. Name three ways your child uses digital technology for education.

   a. _____

   b. _____

   c. _____

23. Name three ways your tween/teen uses digital technology for self-expression. *(Ask your tween/teen for help here.)*

   a. _____

   b. _____

   c. _____

   (Examples include Instagram profile, post on Change.org, online art portfolio, Minecraft creation, avatars, customized website.)

24. Ask your child to give three examples of how he or she can be kind online?

   a. _____

   b. _____

   c. _____

   (Examples include standing up for someone who is being bullied, texting a friend who missed school to give homework, congratulating a friend on Facebook who posted about a big accomplishment.)

25. Have you spelled out specific sites that are forbidden in your family? Yes or No

26. If yes, circle all that apply.

   a. Sexist, racist, homophobic sites

   b. Sites that objectify women such as porn sites

    c. Games with extreme violence and MA ratings

    d. Games or sites that require personal information

    e. Games that mock or bully players

    f. Other _____

27. Have you spelled out specific actions that are forbidden in your family? Yes or No

28. If yes, circle all that apply.

    a. Bullying or cyberbullying

    b. Sexting

    c. Forwarding inappropriate comments or pictures that are sent to you

    d. Pretending to be someone else online

    e. Taking credit for others' work

    f. Hacking

    g. Downloading games or sites without parent approval

    h. Selling items online without parent approval

    i. Other _____

29. Have you discussed privacy and safety issues with your child? Yes or No

30. If no, reread this book. If yes, how do you plan to balance privacy concerns with your tween/teen? Circle all that apply.

    a. Will follow on all social media sites but not comment.

    b. Will occasionally check phone and Internet but won't comment unless there is a safety concern.

    c. Will allow tween to have greater independence over time.

    d. Will not intervene in tween/teen's life but will help to manage digital footprint.

    e. If teen/tween wants more privacy, then recommend using real-life communication rather than electronic communication.

31. Will there be consequences for infractions? If yes, circle/check all that apply.

    a. If child breaks where/when rules, then child will lose technology____ Internet____ phone____ for half day.

    b. Child will lose full day of technology____ Internet____ phone____ on second infraction in same week.

    c. Consequences restart each week.

   d. Content violations will result in loss of above technology and a learning lesson such as apology, community service, family service, etc.

   e. Other consequences _____

32. In return for following family guidelines, your children will be able to do which of the following? Circle all that apply.

   a. Will be able to continue using digital technology in their lives

   b. May be able to explore new areas of interest in cyberspace

   c. Will be granted greater levels of responsibility and independence

I have included three sample templates for family technology agreements. You may photocopy them or go to *www.guilford.com/gold-forms* and download templates to use in your family. I would recommend photocopying (or downloading and printing from *www.guilford.com/gold-forms*) the following guidelines and attaching them to the agreement or posting them somewhere in your home.

CYBER BILL OF RIGHTS

- Technology is a privilege, not a right.
- Technology is a tool, not an end point.
- Your digital footprint begins at birth.
- Privacy doesn't exist in cyberspace.
- The "delete" key should be renamed the "archive" key.
- Be kind online.
- Be an upstander, not a bystander.
- Don't share your passwords or personal information.
- Get permission to download or join new games and social media sites.
- Limit technology in the bedroom.
- Don't sleep with your phone.
- Create tech-free family times daily *(parents included!)*.
- Your digital identity should reflect your true identity.

From *Screen-Smart Parenting*. Copyright 2015 by The Guilford Press.

Good luck in your cyber journey!

Family Digital Technology Agreement: Grades 2–5

Family name _____ Date _____

Our family recognizes that technology is an important part of our lives. We believe that it should be used safely as a tool for organizing, learning, creating, communicating, and fun.

When I can use technology?

- Technology may be used on weekday mornings when the following is completed:
  - Get dressed and gather belongings
  - Eat breakfast
  - Brush teeth
  - Other _____
- Technology may be used after school when the following is completed:
  - After-school activities
  - Homework and chores
  - Playdates
  - Other _____
- Technology may be used on weekends at times specified by parents.
- Technology must be turned off by 8:00 P.M. on weekdays and 9:00 P.M. on weekends.

Where can I use technology?

- No technology in the bedroom.
- Games and Internet in the kitchen, basement, or den.
- Online homework must be done in a common area.
- Technology may be used in the car when car trips exceed 30 minutes.

What I should do online?

- I will occasionally show my parents what I am doing or creating online.
- I will keep my passwords private and share them only with my parents.
- I will not share personal information such as my whole name, address, and birthdate.
- I will look for games and sites that help me learn and explore.

(continued)

- I understand that I can't believe everything I read online.
- I will remember that technology is only one part of my life.

Who do I want to be online?
- I agree to be kind online and to tell my parents if someone is mean to me.
- I agree to tell my parents about anything that makes me uncomfortable.
- I agree not to take credit for others' work online.
- I agree to be an upstander, not a bystander.

What if?
- If I use technology at inappropriate times or inappropriate ways, I will lose all technology for half a day in that given week.
- The second time will result in losing technology for one entire day.
- I agree to tell my parents if my online activities make me feel uncomfortable in any way.

My parents agree:
- To allow me to use digital technology if it is done safely and within the family guidelines.
- To help me find new games, sites, and programs to further explore my interests.
- To listen to my concerns before setting limits and guidelines.
- To recognize that everyone makes mistakes. My parents need to be involved in helping me learn from my mistakes.
- Not to criticize or punish me when I go to them in need.
- To acknowledge that safety and comfort are the top priority.
- To give me more freedom and responsibility with continued safe use.

_____   _____   _____
Child's signature   *Child #2*   *Child #3*

_____   _____
Parent #1 signature   *Parent #2*

_____   _____
Parent #3   *Parent #4*

_____
Date

Family Digital Technology Agreement: Grades 6–8

Family name _____   Date _____

Our family recognizes that technology is an integral part of our lives. We believe that it should be used safely as a tool for organization, learning, creativity, communication, self-expression, and fun.

When I can use technology?

- Technology may be used on weekday mornings when the following is completed:
  - Get dressed and gather belongings
  - Eat breakfast
  - Brush teeth
  - Other _____
- Technology may be used after school when the following is completed:
  - After-school activities
  - Homework and chores
  - Other _____
- My phone needs to be given to an adult from 5:00 to 7:00 P.M. or when my homework is being done.
- I agree to block pop-ups and not surf the Internet or text during homework.
- Technology may be used on weekends after homework is completed. It should not interfere with extracurricular activities, reading, and friend and family activities.
- Technology must be turned off by _____ (suggested 8:30–9:30) P.M. on weekdays and _____ (suggested 10:00–11:30) P.M. on weekends.

Where I can use technology?

- I will not keep my phone or other technology in my bedroom.
- Games and Internet must be used in common areas.
- I will leave my phone in the kitchen charger at bedtime.
- Technology may be used in the car when car trips exceed 30 minutes.

(continued)

What should I do online?

- My parents will occasionally check my texts and Internet.
- My parents will occasionally ask for a tour of my Internet activity.
- I will not share my passwords with anyone other than my parents.
- I will not share personal information online.
- I will join social networks or online games only with my parents' permission.
- I agree not to visit sexist, racist, or homophobic sites.
- I agree to use technology for education and creativity as much as possible.

Who do I want to be online?

- I agree to the tenets of digital citizenship (see attached bill of rights).
- I agree to be kind online.
- I agree to tell my parents about anything that makes me uncomfortable.
- I agree to use technology to present my true self and as a tool for creative expression.
- I agree not to take credit for anyone else's work.
- I agree not to pretend to be anyone else online or to lie about my age.
- I agree not to cyberbully or sext and to tell my parents about any concerns regarding bullying or sexuality.

What if?

- If I use technology at inappropriate times or in inappropriate ways, I will lose my phone for half a day in that given week.
- The second infraction will result in losing my phone for one entire day.
- My parents will always give me a "free pass" from punishment if I go to them with concerns about bullying, sexting, or privacy.
- I agree to tell my parents if my online activities make me feel uncomfortable in any way.

My parents agree:

- To allow me to use digital technology if it is done safely and within the family guidelines.
- To help me find new ways for technology to enhance my life.
- To listen to my concerns before setting limits and guidelines.

(continued)

- To recognize that everyone makes mistakes. My parents need to be involved in helping me to learn from my mistakes.
- Not to criticize or punish me when I come to them in need.
- To acknowledge that safety and comfort are the top priority.
- To advance my independent use with my continued responsible use.
- Throughout high school, my parents will continue to help me monitor my digital footprint.

_____   _____   _____
Child's signature   *Child #2*   *Child #3*

_____   _____
Parent #1 signature   *Parent #2*

_____   _____
Parent #3   *Parent #4*

_____
Date

Family Digital Technology Agreement: High School

Family name _____ Date _____

Our family recognizes that technology is an integral part of our lives. We believe that it should be used safely as a tool for organization, learning, creativity, communication, self-expression, and fun.

When can I use technology?

- My phone should be given to an adult or put in another room when I am doing homework.
- I agree to block pop-ups and not surf the Internet or text during homework.
- I may use technology during the weekend. I recognize that I must find a balance between my real-life obligations and my online activities. Technology should not interfere with extracurricular activities, reading, or friend or family activities.
- I will turn off technology by _____ (suggest 9:30–10:30 P.M. on weekdays) and by _____ (suggested 11:30 P.M.–1:00 A.M. on weekends).

Where can I use technology?

- I will not use technology in my bedroom.
- I will use technology in common areas as much as possible.
- I will leave my phone in the kitchen charger at bedtime.
- I will not text while driving.
- I will use a headset if I need to talk on the phone while driving.
- I will use a car GPS and not a smartphone navigation system.

What should I do online?

- My parents will occasionally check my texts and Internet history.
- Occasionally, I will share my online activities with my parents.
- I must share passwords with my parents.
- I will not share passwords with anyone other than my parents.
- I will make my parents aware of all my active social media sites.
- I agree not to visit sexist, racist, or homophobic sites.

(continued)

- I agree not to meet online friends in person without my parents' permission.
- I agree to use technology for education, creativity, and self-expression as much as possible.

Who do I want to be online?

- I agree to the Cyber Bill of Rights (*see attached*).
- I agree to be kind online and not cyberbully.
- I agree to tell my parents if my online activities make me feel uncomfortable.
- I agree to use technology to present my true self.
- I agree not to take credit for anyone else's work.
- I agree not to pretend to be anyone else online or to lie about my age.
- I agree not to sext.

What if?

- If I use technology at inappropriate times or in inappropriate ways, I will lose my phone for half a day in that given week.
- The second infraction will result in losing my phone for one entire day.
- If I use poor judgment in managing my digital citizenship or digital footprint, I will lose phone privileges and will be asked to find a consequence that can help me learn from my mistakes.
- My parents will always give me a "free pass" from punishment if I go to them with concerns about bullying, sexting, or privacy.
- I agree to tell my parents if my online activities make me feel worse in any way.

My parents agree:

- To allow me to use digital technology if it is done safely and within the family guidelines.
- To help me find new ways for technology to enhance my life.
- To listen to my concerns before setting limits and guidelines.
- To follow me on my social media sites but not comment unless I give them explicit permission.
- To recognize that everyone makes mistakes. My parents need to be involved in helping me to learn from my mistakes.
- Not to criticize or punish me when I come to them in need.

(continued)

- To acknowledge that safety and comfort are the top priority.
- To advance my independent use with my continued responsible use.
- To help me monitor my digital footprint throughout high school.

_____   _____
Teenager's signature   *Teen #2*

_____
Teen #3

_____   _____
Parent #1 signature   *Parent #2*

_____   _____
Parent #3   *Parent #4*

_____
Date

Resources

WEBSITES

General Recommendations and Information

United States

American Academy of Pediatrics (AAP)
SafetyNet
http://safetynet.aap.org
Provides resources and education on safety and growing up online.

Bright Futures
http://brightfutures.aap.org/about.html
AAP's child health and development website with lots of educational materials and assessments.

Centers for Disease Control and Prevention (CDC)
cdc.gov/ncbddd/childdevelopment/facts.html
Offers very detailed information on health, development, and parenting.

National Center for Missing and Exploited Children
NetSmartz Workshop
www.netsmartz.org/InternetSafety

Children's Technology Review
https://childrenstech.com

A subscriber-supported database of children's interactive media products. Products are carefully reviewed and site boasts extensive reviewing guidelines and interrater reliability. Receive monthly newsletters and apps of the week.

Common Sense Media
www.commonsensemedia.org

Nonprofit organization that rates movies, games, and websites. They provide extensive education materials for parents and teachers. Their blog is also a wonderful way to keep up with your child's digital life.

PBS Parents
Child Development
www.pbs.org/parents/child-development

Offers very simplified but thoughtful insights into development.

Children and Media
www.pbs.org/parents/childrenandmedia

Interactive and educational.

Federal Trade Commission (FTC)
Living Life Online
www.consumer.ftc.gov/features/feature-0026-living-life-online

You can order free copies of this manual for ages 8–12.

Admongo.gov

The FTC's attempt to educate kids ages 8–12 specifically about advertising.

You Are Here
www.consumer.ftc.gov/sites/default/files/games/off-site/youarehere/index.html

The FTC's "virtual mall" where kids can play games, design ads, and become smart consumers.

Canada and the United Kingdom

Canadian Paediatric Society
www.cps.ca

Promotes health of children and teens.

Caring for Kids

www.caringforkids.cps.ca/handouts/behaviour-index

General information on health, wellness, and development.

Mediasmarts.ca

Canada's center for digital and media literacy. Provides support and lesson plans for teachers.

KidsandMedia UK

http://kidsandmedia.co.uk

The British site of Kids and Media, a nonprofit organization devoted to giving information and advice about children's use of digital media. Its vision is to see children and teenagers using media with safety and awareness.

Ofcom

www.ofcom.org.uk

The independent regulator for the United Kingdom's communication industries. Offers advice and information for parents, research on children's media use, and more.

Cyberbullying

Stopbullying.gov

Website run by U.S. Department of Health and Human Services.

ThatsNotCool.com

A public education campaign that uses digital examples of controlling, pressuring, and threatening behavior to raise awareness and prevent teen dating abuse. Teens can set up an avatar and create "calling cards" to respond to "pic pressure." Other topics include text harassment, privacy problems, constant messaging, and rumors.

BOOKS

General Child Development

Brazelton, T. Berry. *Touchpoints: Birth to Three*. Da Capo Press. 2006.
Brazelton, T. Berry. *Touchpoints: Three to Six*. Da Capo Press. 2002.
Faber, Adele, & Elaine Mazlish. *How to Talk So Kids Will Listen and Listen So Kids Will Talk*. Scribner. Updated edition. 2012.
Faber, Adele, & Elaine Mazlish. *How to Talk So Teens Will Listen and Listen So Teens Will Talk*. William Morrow Paperbacks. Reprint Edition. 2006.

Faber, Adele, & Elaine Mazlish. *Siblings Without Rivalry: How to Help Your Children Live Together So You Can Live Too.* Norton. 2012.

Fraiberg, Selma. *The Magic Years: Understanding and Handling the Problems of Early Childhood.* Scribner. 1996.—Classic description of the inner lives of young children.

Healy, Jane. *Your Child's Growing Mind: Brain Development and Learning from Birth to Adolescence.* Harmony. 2004.

Karp, Harvey. *The Happiest Toddler on the Block: How to Eliminate Tantrums and Raise a Patient, Respectful, and Cooperative One- to Four-Year-Old.* Random House. Revised edition. 2008.—Very practical and helpful parenting book for new parents.

Mooney, Carol Garhart. *Theories of Attachment: An Introduction to Bowlby, Ainsworth, Gerber, Brazelton, Kennell, and Klaus.* Redleaf Press. 2009.

Mooney, Carol Garhart. *Theories of Childhood: An Introduction to Dewey, Montessori, Erikson, Piaget, and Vygotsky.* Redleaf Press. Second edition. 2013.

Pruitt, David. *Your Child: Emotional, Behavioral, and Cognitive Development from Birth through Preadolescence,* Volume 1. HarperCollins. 2009.

Pruitt, David. *Your Adolescent: Emotional, Behavioral, and Cognitive Development from Early Adolescence through the Teen Years,* Volume 2. HarperCollins. 2009.—This series was sponsored by the American Academy of Child and Adolescent Psychiatry. It gives you a basic overview of milestones and development.

Tough, Paul. *How Children Succeed: Grit, Curiosity, and the Hidden Power of Character.* Mariner Books. Reprint 2013.—Well-written and -researched book that explores the topic of raising kids with resilience.

Parenting and Digital Media

Edgington, Shawn Marie. *The Parent's Guide to Texting, Facebook, and Social Media: Understanding the Benefits and Dangers of Parenting in a Digital World.* Brown Books Publishing Group. 2011.

Steyer, James P. *Talking Back to Facebook: The Common Sense Guide to Raising Kids in the Digital Age.* Scribner. 2012.

Summers, Patti Wollman, Ann DeSollar-Hale, & Heather Ibrahim-Leathers. *Toddlers on Technology: A Parents' Guide.* AuthorHouse. 2013.

ADHD, Anxiety, and Depression in Children and Adolescents

Barkley, Russell A. *Taking Charge of ADHD: The Complete, Authoritative Guide for Parents.* Guilford Press. Third edition. 2013.

Greene, Ross W. *The Explosive Child: A New Approach for Understanding and Parenting Easily Frustrated, Chronically Inflexible Children.* Harper Paperbacks. Revised edition. 2010.

Last, Cynthia G. *Help for Worried Kids: How Your Child Can Conquer Anxiety and Fear.* Guilford Press. 2006.

Oster, Gerald D., & Sarah S. Montgomery. *Helping Your Depressed Teenager: A Guide for Parents and Caregivers.* Wiley. 1994.

Reiff, Michael I. *ADHD: What Every Parent Needs to Know.* American Academy of Pediatrics. Second edition. 2011.

Schaefer, Charles E., & Theresa Foy DiGeronimo. *Ages & Stages: A Parent's Guide to Normal Childhood Development.* Wiley. 2000.

Seligman, Martin. *The Optimistic Child: A Proven Program to Safeguard Children against Depression and Build Lifelong Resilience.* Mariner Books. Reprint edition. 2007.

Spencer, Elizabeth DuPont, Robert L. DuPont, & Caroline M. DuPont. *The Anxiety Cure for Kids: A Guide for Parents and Children.* Wiley. Second edition. 2014.

Notes

CHAPTER 1

1. David Dobbs, "The Science of Success," *Atlantic Monthly*, December 2009, *http://www.theatlantic.com/magazine/archive/2009/12/the-science-of-success/307761*.

2. Leen d'Haenens, Sofie Vandoninick, and Veronica Donoso, "How to Cope and Build Online Resilience," EU Kids Online, January 2013, *www.lse.ac.uk/media@lse/research/EUKidsOnline/EU%20Kids%20III/Reports/Copingonlineresilience.pdf*. Findings are based on an in-home face-to-face survey of 25,000 kids ages 9–16 in 25 European countries. This study also addresses coping strategies.

3. Paul Tough, *How Children Succeed: Grit, Curiosity, and the Hidden Power of Character* (New York: Houghton Mifflin Harcourt, 2012). Highly recommended for an understanding of the research behind character and a new approach to education.

4. The details of E-rate grants and CIPA are complicated. The Universal Service Administrative Company (USAC) provides application information at *www.usac.org/sl*. I found the Elk Grove Unified School District blog to be most helpful in explaining the digital citizenship requirements for school districts (*http://blogs.egusd.net/digitalcitizenship*).

5. Mathew S. Eastin, Bradley S. Greenberg, and Linda Hofschire, "Parenting the Internet," *Journal of Communication* 56 (2006): 486–504. The article cites studies for each of these measures.

6. Martin Valcke, Sarah Bonte, Bram De Wever, and Isabel Rots, "Internet Parenting Styles and the Impact on Internet Use of Primary School Children," *Computers & Education* 55, no. 2 (2010): 454–64. Good overview of general parenting styles and how parenting style can affect a child's digital life.

7. Ellen Wartella, Victoria Rideout, Alexis R. Lauricella, and Sabrina L.

Connell, *Parenting in the Age of Digital Technology: A National Survey*, Center on Media and Human Development, School of Communication, Northwestern University, June 2013, *http://vjrconsulting.com/storage/PARENTING_IN_THE_AGE_OF_DIGITAL_TECHNOLOGY.pdf*, pp. 1–30.

8. Victoria Rideout, Ulla G. Foehr, and Donald Roberts, *Generation M2: Media in the Lives of 8- to 18-Year-Olds* (Menlo Park, CA: Kaiser Family Foundation, 2010). This is the most exhaustive and highly referenced study of media usage in the United States.

CHAPTER 2

1. Genevieve Johnson, "Internet Use and Cognitive Development: A Theoretical Framework," *E-Learning and Digital Media* 3, no. 4 (2006): 565–73.

2. Ibid., 565–67.

3. Russell M. Viner and Tim J. Cole, "Television Viewing in Early Childhood Predicts Adult Body Mass Index," *Journal of Pediatrics* 147, no. 4 (2005): 429–35.

4. John J. Reilly, Julie Armstrong, Ahmad R. Dorosty, Pauline Emmett, A. Ness, I. Rogers, et al., "Early Life Risk Factors for Obesity in Childhood: Cohort Study," *British Medical Journal* 330, no. 7504 (2005): 1357.

5. Victoria Rideout, Ulla G. Foehr, and Donald Roberts, *Generation M2: Media in the Lives of 8- to 18-Year-Olds* (Menlo Park, CA: Kaiser Family Foundation, 2010); Ellen Wartella, Victoria Rideout, Alexis R. Lauricella, and Sabrina L. Connell, *Parenting in the Age of Digital Technology: A National Survey*, Center on Media and Human Development, School of Communication, Northwestern University, June 2013, *http://vjrconsulting.com/storage/PARENTING_IN_THE_AGE_OF_DIGITAL_TECHNOLOGY.pdf*, pp. 1–30.

6. Barbara A. Dennison, Tara A. Erb, and Paul L. Jenkins, "Television Viewing and Television in Bedroom Associated with Overweight Risk among Low-Income Preschool Children," *Pediatrics* 109, no. 6 (2002): 1028–35; Daheia J. Barr-Anderson, Patricia van den Berg, Dianne Neumark-Sztainer, and Mary Story, "Characteristics Associated with Older Adolescents Who Have a Television in Their Bedrooms," *Pediatrics* 121, no. 4 (2008): 718–24.

7. Anna M. Adachi-Mejia, Meghan R. Longacre, Lucinda Gibson, Michael L. Beach, Linda Titus-Ernstoff , and Madeline A. Dalton, "Children with a TV Set in Their Bedroom at Higher Risk for Being Overweight," *International Journal of Obesity* 31, no. 4 (2007): 644–51.

8. Victor C. Strasburger and the Council on Communications and Media, American Academy of Pediatrics, "Children, Adolescents, Obesity, and the Media," *Pediatrics* 128, no. 1 (2011): 201–8. Policy paper provides good overview of obesity data.

9. Diana L. Graf, Lauren V. Pratt, Casey N. Hester, and Kevin R. Short, "Playing Active Video Games Increases Energy Expenditure in Children," *Pediatrics* 124, no. 2 (2009): 534–40.

10. Rideout et al., *Generation M2*; Wartella et al., *Parenting in the Age of Digital Technology*.

11. Victor C. Strasburger, Amy Jordan, and Ed Donnerstein, "Health Effects of Media on Children and Adolescents," *Pediatrics* 125, no. 4 (2010): 756–67.

12. Kristen Harrison and Amy L. Marske, "Nutritional Content of Foods Advertised during the Television Programs Children Watch Most," *American Journal of Public Health* 95, no. 9 (2005): 1568–74.

13. Carmen Stitt and Dale Kunkel, "Food Advertising during Children's Television Programming on Broadcast and Cable Channels," *Health Communication* 23, no. 6 (2008): 573–84.

14. Walter Gantz, Nancy Schwartz, James R. Angelini, and Victoria Rideout, *Food for Thought: Television Food Advertising to Children in the United States* (Menlo Park, CA: Kaiser Family Foundation, 2007).

15. Thomas N. Robinson, Dina L. G. Borzekowski, Donna M. Mathesan, and Helena C. Kraemer, "Effects of Fast Food Branding on Young Children's Taste Preferences," *Archives of Pediatrics and Adolescent Medicine* 161, no. 8 (2007): 792–97.

16. Lisa Anne Matricciani, Tim S. Olds, Sarah Blunden, Gabrielle Rigney, and Marie T. Willias, "Never Enough Sleep: A Brief History of Sleep Recommendations for Children," *Pediatrics* 129, no. 3 (2012): 548–56.

17. Neralie Cain and Michael Gradisar, "Electronic Media Use and Sleep in School-Aged Children and Adolescents: A Review," *Sleep Medicine* 11, no. 8 (2010): 735–42.

18. Natalie D. Barlett, Douglas A. Gentile, Christopher P. Barlett, Joey C. Eisenmann, and David A. Walsh, "Sleep as a Mediator of Screen Time Effects on U.S. Children's Health Outcomes," special issue, *Journal of Children and Media* 6, no. 1 (2012): 37–50.

19. Stephani Sutherland, "Bright Lights Could Delay Bedtime," *Scientific American* 23, no. 6, December 19, 2012, *http://www.scientificamerican.com/article/bright-screens-could-delay-bedtime*.

20. Shenghui Li, Xinming Jin, Shenguhu Wu, Fan Jiang, Chonghuai Yan, and Xiaoming Shen, "The Impact of Media Use on Sleep Patterns and Sleep Disorders among School-Aged Children in China," *Sleep* 30, no. 3 (2007): 361–67.

21. Harneet Chahal, Christina Fung, Stefan Kuhle, and Paul J. Veugelers, "Availability and Night-Time Use of Electronic Entertainment and Communication Devices Are Associated with Short Sleep Duration and Obesity among Canadian Children," *Pediatric Obesity* 8, no. 1 (2012): 42–51.

22. Johnson, "Internet Use and Cognitive Development," 570.

23. Patti Wollman Summers, Ann DeSollar-Hale, and Heather Ibrahim-Leathers, *Toddlers on Technology* (Bloomington, IN: AuthorHouse, 2013), 16.

24. Dimitri Christakis, Healthy Media Use, Seattle Children's Hospital, 2009, *https://www.seattlechildrens.org/healthcare-professionals/aar/2009/highlights/healthy-media-use/*.

25. Moses, A. M., "Impacts of Television Viewing on Young Children's Literacy Development in the USA: A Review of the Literature," *Journal of Early Childhood Literacy* 8, no. 1 (2008): 67–102.

26. Johnson, "Internet Use and Cognitive Development."

27. Fran C. Blumberg and Lori M. Sokol, "Boys' and Girls' Use of Cognitive Strategy When Learning to Play Video Games," *Journal of General Psychology* 131, no. 2 (2004): 151–58.

28. Nicholas Carr, *The Shallows: What the Internet Is Doing to Our Brains* (New York: Norton, 2010), 7–20.

29. I. Sharif and J. D. Sargent, "Association Between Television, Movie, and Video Game Exposure and School Performance." *Pediatrics* 118, no. 4 (2006), e1061–e1070.

30. Patti M. Valkenburg and Jochen Peter, "Online Communication and Adolescent Well-Being: Testing the Stimulation versus the Displacement Hypothesis," *Journal of Computer-Mediated Communication* 12, no. 4 (2007): 1169–82.

31. Elise Clerkin, April Smith, and Jennifer L. Hames, "Interpersonal Effects of Facebook Reassurance Seeking," *Journal of Affective Disorders* 151, no. 2 (2013): 525–29.

CHAPTER 3

1. Poynter.org Provides very good glossary for journalists writing about technology.

2. Victoria Rideout, Ulla G. Foehr, and Donald Roberts, *Generation M2: Media in the Lives of 8- to 18-Year-Olds* (Menlo Park, CA: Kaiser Family Foundation, 2010), 3.

3. Ibid., 33–34.

4. Ibid., 15–17.

5. Statistics for YouTube and Netflix from "Top 15 Most Popular Video Websites, May 2014," eBizMBA website, *www.ebizmba.com/articles/video-websites*.

6. Elizabeth Englander, "Research Findings: MARC 2011 Survey Grades 3–12," *MARC Research Reports*, Paper 2, Bridgewater State University, 2011, *http://cdn.theatlantic.com/static/mt/assets/science/Research%20Findings_%20MARC%20 2011%20Survey%20Grades%203-12.pdf.*

7. Shawn Marie Edgington, *The Parent's Guide to Texting, Facebook, and Social Media: Understanding the Benefits and Dangers of Parenting in a Digital World* (Dallas, TX: Brown Books, 2011), 19 (includes all three per-month statistics).

8. Rideout et al., *Generation M2*, 18.

9. Hara Estroff Marano, "A Nation of Wimps," *Psychology Today*, November 2004, *www.psychologytoday.com/articles/200411/nation-wimps*.

10. Rideout et al., *Generation M2*.

11. Ibid., 22.

12. Most of the details about video games come from Wikipedia, online blogs, and interviews with more experienced gamers.

13. I tried to piece together a general outline of the video game devices and genres from Wikipedia, online dictionaries, and video game blogs.

14. Jane McGonigal, "Be a Gamer, Save the World," *Wall Street Journal*, January 22, 2011.

15. Ellen Wartella, Victoria Rideout, Alexis R. Lauricella, and Sabrina L. Connell, *Parenting in the Age of Digital Technology: A National Survey*, Center on Media and Human Development, School of Communication, Northwestern University, June 2013, *http://vjrconsulting.com/storage/PARENTING_IN_THE_AGE_OF_DIGITAL_TECHNOLOGY.pdf.*

16. Jane McGonigal, *Reality Is Broken: Why Games Make Us Better and How They Can Change the World* (New York: Penguin, 2011).

17. "Facebook Is Still a Must for American Teens," Statista website, from a 2012 Pew Research Center study, on social media and teens. In 2012 Facebook had the most teen and young adult users (12–24 years). This has changed with each season. Twitter took mantle in 2013 and Instagram in 2014. It looks like Snapchat may be a big rival in 2015. *www.marketingcharts.com/wp/online/instagram-now-tops-twitter-facebook-as-teens-most-important-social-network-41924/.*

Snapchat Seen More Popular than Twitter Among 12–24-Year-Olds. *www.marketingcharts.com/wp/online/snapchat-seen-more-popular-than-twitter-among-12-24-year-olds-41252/.* Research done by Piper Jaffray market research firm.

18. Kelly Schryver, "11 Sites and Apps Kids Are Heading to After Facebook," blog post, Common Sense Media, September 20, 2013, *www.commonsensemedia.org/blog/11-sites-and-apps-kids-are-heading-to-after-facebook#Tumblr.*

CHAPTER 4

1. Shannan Yangar, "Yik Yak App Is Wreaking Havoc in Schools: 11 Things Parents Need to Know," *Tween Us* blog post, March 4, 2014, *www.chicagonow.com/tween-us/2014/03/yik-yak-app-parents-need-to-know.*

2. Victoria Rideout, Ulla G. Foehr, and Donald Roberts, *Generation M2: Media in the Lives of 8- to 18-Year-Olds* (Menlo Park, CA: Kaiser Family Foundation, 2010).

3. Modified from the popular meme "Being Famous on Facebook Is Like Being Rich in Monopoly." *http://memecrunch.com/meme/11QA1/being-famous-on-instagram-is-like-being-rich-in-monopoly.*

4. Clare Wood, Sally Meachem, Samantha Bowyer, Emma Jackson, M. Luisa Tarczynski-Bowles, and Beverly Plester, "A Longitudinal Study of Children's Text Messaging and Literacy Development," *British Journal of Psychology* 102 (2011): 431–42.

5. Jocelyn Glei, "10 Online Tools for Better Attention and Focus," *http://99u.com/articles/6969/10-online-tools-for-better-attention-focus.*

CHAPTER 5

1. Adam Gopnik, excerpt from "Bumping into Mr. Ravioli," *The New Yorker*, September 30, 2002.

2. Ellen Wartella, Victoria Rideout, Alexis R. Lauricella, and Sabrina L. Connell, *Parenting in the Age of Digital Technology: A National Survey*, Center on Media

and Human Development, School of Communication, Northwestern University, June 2013, *http://vjrconsulting.com/storage/PARENTING_IN_THE_AGE_OF_DIGITAL_TECHNOLOGY.pdf*, p. 24. The Northwestern study reports one hour and 15 minutes, with 59 minutes on TV. The Common Sense Media study cited in note 3 below reports 44 minutes. Fair to say approximately 1 hour on media.

3. "Zero to Eight: Children's Media Use in America 2013," Common Sense Media Research Study, *https://www.commonsensemedia.org/research/zero-to-eight-childrens-media-use-in-america-2013*.

4. "Children, Adolescents, and the Media," policy statement, American Academy of Pediatrics, *Pediatrics* 132, no. 5 (November 2013): 958–61, *http://pediatrics.aappublications.org/content/132/5/958.abstract?rss=1*.

5. David L. Hill, "Why to Avoid TV before Age 2," HealthyChildren.org, American Academy of Pediatrics, May 11, 2013, *www.healthychildren.org/english/family-life/media/pages/why-to-avoid-tv-before-age-2.aspx*.

6. Christopher J. Ferguson and M. Brent Donnellan, "Is the Association between Children's Baby Video Viewing and Poor Language Development Robust?: A Reanalysis of Zimmerman, Christakis, and Meltzoff (2007)," *Developmental Psychology*, July 15, 2013, *www.christopherjferguson.com/BabyVideos.pdf*.

7. I found the most thoroughly researched and referenced summary on Wikipedia, at *wikipedia.org/wiki/Baby_Einstein*.

CHAPTER 6

1. Selma Fraiberg, *The Magic Years: Understanding and Handling the Problems of Early Childhood* (New York: Scribner, 1996). This is the best book to give you an understanding of the world of a toddler.

2. Ellen Wartella, Victoria Rideout, Alexis R. Lauricella, and Sabrina L. Connell, *Parenting in the Age of Digital Technology: A National Survey*, Center on Media and Human Development, School of Communication, Northwestern University, June 2013, *http://vjrconsulting.com/storage/PARENTING_IN_THE_AGE_OF_DIGITAL_TECHNOLOGY.pdf*, p. 24.

3. Ibid.

4. Patti Wollman Summers, Ann DeSollar-Hale, and Heather Ibrahim-Leathers, *Toddlers on Technology* (Bloomington, IN: AuthorHouse, 2013), 12–18.

5. Marjorie Hogan, "Prosocial Effects of Media," *Pediatric Clinics of North America* 59, no. 3 (2012): 635–45.

6. Cynthia Chiong, Jinny Ree, Lori Takeuchi, and Ingrid Erickson, *Print Books vs. E-books: Comparing Parent-Child Co-reading on Print, Basic and Enhanced E-book Platforms*, report, the Joan Ganz Cooney Center, spring 2012, *www.joanganzcooneycenter.org/wp-content/uploads/2012/07/jgcc_ebooks_quickreport.pdf*.

CHAPTER 7

1. Ellen Wartella, Victoria Rideout, Alexis R. Lauricella, and Sabrina L. Connell, *Parenting in the Age of Digital Technology: A National Survey*, Center on

Media and Human Development, School of Communication, Northwestern University, June 2013, *http://vjrconsulting.com/storage/PARENTING_IN_THE_AGE_OF_DIGITAL_TECHNOLOGY.pdf*, p. 7–8.

2. Ibid., p. 7–8.

3. Lisa Guernsey, Michael Levine, Cynthia Chiong, and Maggie Severns, "Pioneering Literacy in the Digital Wild West: Empowering Parents and Educators," Joan Ganz Cooney Center, 2012, *www.joanganzcooneycenter.org/wp-content/uploads/2012/12/GLR_TechnologyGuide_final.pdf*.

4. "Minecraft: Construction and Destruction in Equal Measure," review, CVG website, January 14, 2012, *www.computerandvideogames.com/331531/reviews/minecraft-review/#future*.

5. Keith Stuart, "Minecraft at 33 Million Users: A Personal Story," *Guardian*, September 5, 2013.

CHAPTER 8

1. Victoria Rideout, Ulla G. Foehr, and Donald Roberts, *Generation M2: Media in the Lives of 8- to 18-Year-Olds* (Menlo Park, CA: Kaiser Family Foundation, 2010). This is the most exhaustive study looking at 8- to 18-year-olds. It is updated every 5 years so they have been able to track the changes in usage since 1999.

2. Ibid.

3. Ibid.

4. "Super Digital Citizen (3–5)," lesson plan, Common Sense Media, *www.commonsensemedia.org/educators/lesson/super-digital-citizen-3–5*.
Common Sense Media's Scope and Sequence curriculum has downloadable lesson plans that cover topics such as digital footprint, privacy, relationships, self-image, literacy, cyberbullying, and creative copyright.

5. Lisa Fogarty, "Teacher's Photo Goes Viral in Brilliant Lesson on the Dangers of Posting Online," *The Stir* (blog), November 27, 2013, *http://thestir.cafemom.com/technology/164774/teachers_photo_goes_viral_in*.

CHAPTER 9

1. Victoria Rideout, Ulla G. Foehr, and Donald Roberts, *Generation M2: Media in the Lives of 8- to 18-Year-Olds* (Menlo Park, CA: Kaiser Family Foundation, 2010).

2. Ibid.

3. Ibid.

4. "Digital Life 101," lesson plan, Common Sense Media, *https://www.commonsensemedia.org/educators/lesson/digital-life-101-6-8*.

5. Janell Burley Hofmann, "Gregory's iPhone Contract," July 8, 2013, *http://www.janellburleyhofmann.com/postjournal/gregorys-iphone-contract/#.U0m57MeHkXx*.

6. Ann Brenoff, "How I Spy on My Kids," *Huffington Post,* March 22, 2013, *huffingtonpost.com/ann-brenoff/spying-on-kids-online_b_2839081.html.*

7. Nicholas Carr, *The Shallows: What the Internet Is Doing to Our Brains* (New York: Norton, 2010).

8. Ben Parr, "The Average Teenager Sends 3,339 Texts per Month," *Mashable,* October 14, 2010, *http://mashable.com/2010/10/14/nielsen-texting-stats.*

9. "U.S. Teen Mobile Report: Calling Yesterday, Texting Today and Using Apps Tomorrow," Nielsen website, October 10, 2014, *http://www.nielsen.com/us/ en/newswire/2010/u-s-teen-mobile-report-calling-yesterday-texting-today-using-apps-tomorrow.html.*

10. Shawn Marie Edgington, *The Parent's Guide to Texting, Facebook, and Social Media: Understanding the Benefits and Dangers of Parenting in a Digital World* (Dallas, TX: Brown Books, 2011), 20.

11. Scott Frank, Laura Santurri, and Kristina Knight, *Hyper-Texting and Hyper-Networking: A New Health Risk Category for Teens?* School of Medicine, Case Western Reserve University, 2010, *http://www.jjie.org/wp-content/uploads/2010/11/ Hyper-Texting-Study.pdf.*

12. Edgington, *Texting, Facebook, and Social Media,* xiii-xviii. Discusses Megan Meier's suicide and Edgington's campaign to address cyberbullying.

13. Lenhart, A., "Cyberbullying and Online Teens," Pew Internet & American Life Project, June 27, 2007, *www.pewinternet.org.* 2007 study found prevalence rates to be age and gender specific, ranging from 22 to 41%.

14. Cyberbullying Research Center conducted a review of cyberbullying research and found prevalence rates to be approximate 25%. *http://cyberbullying. us/research/facts/.* See section "Cyberbullying Trends and Recent Data."

15. Statistics on missed school days due to bullying are murky. The most commonly cited statistic is that 160,000 kids miss school each day due to bullying. While widely reported, it is a figure from the 1990s that may not be accurate today.

16. Eleanor Barkhorn, "160,000 Kids Stay Home Each Day to Avoid Being Bullied," *Atlantic,* October 3, 2013, *www.theatlantic.com/education/ archive/2013/10/160–000-kids-stay-home-from-school-each-day-to-avoid-being-bullied/280201.*

CHAPTER 10

1. Victoria Rideout, Ulla G. Foehr, and Donald Roberts, *Generation M2: Media in the Lives of 8- to 18-Year-Olds* (Menlo Park, CA: Kaiser Family Foundation, 2010).

2. Amanda Lenhart, Mary Madden, Aaron Smith, Kristin Purcell, Kathryn Zickuhr, and Lee Rainie, "Teens, Kindness and Cruelty on Social Network Sites: How American Teens Navigate the New World of Digital Citizenship," Pew Research Center, Internet and American Life Project, November 9, 2011, *www. pewinternet.org/2011/11/09/teens-kindness-and-cruelty-on-social-network-sites.*

3. Emily Cohn, "LinkedIn Opens Floodgates to Teens with Launch

of University Pages," *Huffington Post,* August 19, 2013, *www.huffingtonpost. com/2013/08/19/linkedin-teenagers-university-pages_n_3776504.html.*

4. "Teens and Social Media: Young People Who Used the Internet To Do Major Good, *HuffPost Teen,* June 26, 2013, *www.huffingtonpost.com/2013/06/26/teens-using-social-media_n_3505564.html.*

5. Krystie Yandoli, "High School Students Build Car Fueled by Twitter, Facebook and Other Social Media," *Huffington Post,* May 24, 2013, *www. huffingtonpost.com/2013/05/24/high-school-students-buil_1_n_3333068.html.*

6. Emma Penrod, "Teen Activists Combat Body Image Negativity with Online Tools," *Deseret News,* July 4, 2013 (national edition).

7. *Oxford Dictionaries* online, *http://blog.oxforddictionaries.com/2013/11/word-of-the-year-2013-winner.*

8. "Dove Short Film Embraces 'Selfies' to Redefine How We Perceive Beauty," *http://mashable.com/2014/01/20/dove-selfies-short-film.*

9. Lauren A. Jelenchick, Jens C. Eickhoff, and Megan A. Moreno, "Facebook Depression? Social Networking Site Use and Depression in Older Adolescents," *Journal of Adolescent Health* 52, no. 1 (2013): 128–30.

10. Ethan Kross, Philippe Verduyn, Emre Demiralp, Jiyoung Park, David Seungjae Lee, Natalie Lin, et al., "Facebook Use Predicts Declines in Subjective Well-Being in Young Adults," *PLoS ONE* 8, no. 8 (2013): e69841.

11. Corey J. Blomfield Neira and Bonnie L. Barber, "Social Networking Site Use Linked to Adolescents' Self-concept, Self-esteem and Depressed Mood," *Australian Journal of Psychology* 66 (2014): 56–64.

12. Association for Family Interactive Media, "Sex and Tech: Results from a Survey of Teens and Young Adults," *www.afim.org/SexTech_Summary.pdf;* Lenhart et al., "Teens, Kindness and Cruelty."

13. Donald S. Strassberg, Ryan K. McKinnon, Michael A. Sustaita, and Jordan Rullo, "Sexting by High School Students: An Exploratory and Descriptive Study," *Archives of Sexual Behavior* 42, no. 1 (2013): 15–21.

14. Jan Hoffman, "A Girl's Nude Photo, and Altered Lives," *New York Times,* March 27, 2011, *www.nytimes.com/2011/03/27/us/27sexting.html?pagewanted=all&_r=0.*

15. Hara Estroff Marano, "A Nation of Wimps," *Psychology Today,* November 2004, *www.psychologytoday.com/articles/200411/nation-wimps.*

16. Lenhart et al., "Teens, Kindness and Cruelty."

17. "What Would Honest Abe Lincoln Say?" Josephson Institute of Ethics, February 10, 2011, *http://charactercounts.org/programs/reportcard/2010/installment02_report-card_honesty-integrity.html.*

CHAPTER 11

1. Stephanie Bioulac, Lisa Arfi, and Manuel P. Bouvard, "Attention Deficit/Hyperactivity Disorder and Video Games: A Comparative Study of Hyperactive and Control Children," *European Psychiatry* 23, no. 2 (2008): 134–41.

2. Ibid.

3. Margaret D. Weiss, Susan Baer, Blake Allan, Kelly Saran, and Heidi Schibuk, "The Screens Culture: Impact on ADHD," *Attention Deficit Hyperactivity Disorder* 3, no. 4 (2011): 327–34.

4. Ibid.

5. Doug Hyun Han, Young Sik Lee, Churl Na, Jee Young Ahn, Un Sun Chung, Melissa A. Daniels, et al., "The Effect of Methylphenidate on Internet Video Game Play in Children with Attention-Deficit/Hyperactivity Disorder," *Comprehensive Psychiatry* 50, no. 3 (2009): 251–56.

6. Luigi Bonetti, Marilyn Anne Campbell, and Linda Gilmore, "The Relationship of Loneliness and Social Anxiety with Children's and Adolescents' Online Communication," *Cyberpsychology, Behavior, and Social Networking* 13, no. 3 (2010): 279–85.

7. Jeffrey P. Harman, Catherine E. Hansen, Margaret E. Cochran, and Cynthia R. Lindsey, "Liar, Liar: Internet Faking But Not Frequency of Use Affects Social Skills, Self-Esteem, Social Anxiety, and Aggression," *Cyberpsychology and Behavior* 8, no. 1 (2005): 1–6.

8. Michaelle Indian and Rachel Grieve, "When Facebook Is Easier Than Face-To-Face: Social Support Derived from Facebook in Socially Anxious Individuals," *Personality and Individual Differences* 59 (2014): 102–6.

9. Patti Valkenburg and Jochen Peter, "Social Consequences of the Internet for Adolescents: A Decade of Research," *Current Directions in Psychological Science* 18, no. 1 (2009): 1–5.

10. "Depression in Children and Adolescents," fact sheet, National Institute of Mental Health, *www.nimh.nih.gov/health/publications/depression-in-children-and-adolescents/depression-in-children-and-adolescents.pdf.*

11. Vladimir Carli, Christina W. Hoven, Camilla Wasserman, Flaminia Chiesa, Guia Guffanti, Marco Sarchiapone, et al., "A Newly Identified Group of Adolescents at "Invisible" Risk for Psychopathology and Suicidal Behavior: Findings from the SEYLE Study," *World Psychiatry* 13, no. 1 (2014): 78–86.

12. Erick Messias, Juan Castro, Anil Saini, Manzoor Usman, and Dale Peeples. "Sadness, Suicide, and Their Association with Video Game and Internet Overuse Among Teens: Results from the Youth Risk Behavior Survey 2007 and 2009," *Suicide Life-Threatening Behavior* 41, no. 3 (2011): 307–15.

13. Sriram Chellappan and Raghavendra Kotikalapudi, "How Depressives Surf the Web," *New York Times*, June 15, 2012, *www.nytimes.com/2012/06/17/opinion/sunday/how-depressed-people-use-the-internet.html?_r=2&pagewanted=all.*

14. Romeo Vitelli, "Suicide and the Internet: Can Online Suicide Sites Increase Suicide Risk?" *Psychology Today*, October 7, 2013.

Index

AB Math, 158
Academics. *See* School and academics
ADHD, 92, 248–256
Adolescents. *See* Teenagers; Tweens
Aggression, 128
Alone Together (Turkle), 50–51
Anti-Social (app), 93
Anxiety. *See* Social anxiety
Apps and games
    for children in the early elementary
        years, 147, 149–150, 156–159
    for toddlers, 126, 130–131, 132
Ask.fm, 74, 78, 82, 254
Attachment theory, 30, 104–105
Attention deficit/hyperactivity disorder.
    See ADHD
Authoritarian parenting, 20, 21
Authoritative parenting, 20–21

B

Babies (ages 0–2)
    cognitive development and, 41–43
    digital technology use, 102
    educational videos and, 108–109
    "good-enough mother" concept, 103
    impact of parents' relationship with
        technology, 112–114
    importance of attachment, 104–105

screen-time recommendations for, 105
siblings' digital technology use and,
    110–112
use of media to babysit, 105–107
Baby Einstein, 108–109
Behavioral plans, 267–270
Body image issues, 180–181
Brain development, 31–32, 41–43, 90–92.
    See also Cognitive development
Brownie Points, 158

C

Cell phones
    developmental approach to children
        acquiring, 77–78
    in the early elementary years, 155–156
    in the late elementary years, 179–180
    overview of core issues, 58–61
    smartphones as educational tools for
        toddlers, 125
    taking away a child's phone, 275–276
    tweens and, 195–196
    See also Texting
Chat, 60
Child development
    cognitive development, 31–32, 40–46.
        See also Cognitive development
    moral development, 140, 163–165

About the Author

Jodi Gold, MD, is a board-certified child and adolescent psychiatrist in private practice and Clinical Assistant Professor at Weill Cornell Medical College. A nationally recognized expert, Dr. Gold speaks, writes, and makes media appearances on her developmental approach to parenting in the age of digital technology. She lives with her husband and three children in New York City.